Overcoming Common Problems Series

Overcoming Common Problems Series

Overcoming Common Problems

TREATING ARTHRITIS
More ways to a drug-free life

Margaret Hills SRN

sheldon **PRESS**

My thanks go to my daughter-in-law, Jane,
for typing this book

First published in Great Britain in 1991

Sheldon Press
36 Causton Street
London SW1P 4ST
www.sheldonpress.co.uk

Reprinted nine times
Re-issued 2008

British Library Cataloguing-in-Publication Data
A catalogue record for this book is available from the British Library

ISBN 978-1-84709-040-9

3 5 7 9 10 8 6 4 2

Typeset by Deltatype Ltd, Birkenhead, Merseyside
Printed in Great Britain by Ashford Colour Press

Produced on paper from sustainable forests

For my children and grandchildren

Contents

Foreword

I have undertaken to publish the story of my experiences at my clinic in Coventry because I feel I can use this opportunity to express my views on sickness and disease and their relationship to natural healing and indeed their relationship to divine healing. It is my belief that all healing comes from God – The Great Healer. I have carried this philosophy with me throughout my life, and no doubt it was planted there by my devout Catholic mother whose words, 'God is good', I shall never forget. In every crisis she used these words, and there were many crises. She was mother of eight children – I was her first born. Times were hard, my father was not a well man, but with God's help they overcame all difficulties and brought up a family to be proud of. I also have eight children, five boys and three girls. I hope that I can give them the same wonderful example that my parents gave their family. They taught us faith, hope, and love for one another, for humanity and most of all for God. I can only speak for myself, but I must say that my parents' example has had a very far reaching effect on my life, and as I go through my consultations day by day I never fail to ask the Lord to help me to heal those he has sent to me for help. I know that without his help there will be no healing.

My first book, *Treating Arthritis – The Drug-Free Way* has helped many people in many countries, and I feel very strongly that this one will give even more hope and encouragement to sufferers of arthritis all over the world.

Margaret Hills
January 1991

Introduction

Having worked for several years with arthritic people in my Coventry clinic, I feel confident that the information presented in this book is ripe for publication. I hope it will be useful for the hundreds of patients I have already treated, and for current patients (approximately 1500 at the last count), and especially for arthritis sufferers who would like to take advantage of our treatment but because they have relatives or friends who are against 'natural' treatment do not contact us.

Fortunately, most General Practitioners are becoming aware of and open to natural treatments. Some have even contacted my clinic for treatment for themselves – and have written to tell us that they are doing well.

Rheumatology consultants in several hospitals have seen a vast improvement in their patients' health and some patients who have spent years taking drugs for arthritis but whose health has still gone steadily down hill, have now got rid of their arthritis altogether and have been discharged from hospital.

I wonder why doctors and consultants do not take more notice of the successes they encounter due to natural treatment. One reason could be that many patients are scared to tell their GPs and consultants that they attend this clinic. I tell them that they should tell their doctors because the doctors and consultants must be very surprised when they see a patient who has been steadily getting worse for years, suddenly doing a U-turn and getting better. Doctors know that drugs for arthritis do not have this effect. As the days go by, and I get more and more reports from my patients about how amazed their doctors and consultants are at their progress, I can't help wondering why these doctors and consultants do not contact me to learn why my patients improve to such an extent that they can dispense with their drugs and lead a normal life. I hope that this book may be read by members of the medical profession so that they can become more aware of my methods and positive results.

This book is organized into five chapters. Chapters 1 and 2

describe how arthritis usually manifests itself, and how it can be treated, in children and adults respectively.

Chapter 3 gives twelve Case Histories, illustrating how patients have been treated, either in person or by post, through the Margaret Hills Clinic. The Case Histories are wonderful reading for anyone starting out on the treatment as they show unfailingly positive results.

Chapter 4 discusses the stress factor, how it affects the body and contributes to arthritis, and how it can be alleviated.

Chapter 5 is an extremely useful and informative list of questions and answers. Anyone wishing to start the treatment would be well advised to read this section thoroughly.

1

Arthritis in Children

In the daily running of my clinic I come into contact with many patients of all ages whose every movement is absolute agony through either rheumatoid or osteoarthritis. These diseases are on the increase amongst young and old alike, and as stated in my previous book, *Curing Arthritis – The Drug-Free Way*, we can lay the blame on the food we eat and the drinks we consume.

Symptoms

Rheumatoid arthritis can manifest itself in the young or old, it affects the coverings of the bones of the joint, gradually causing stiffness. It affects many joints simultaneously or successively. Children suffering from rheumatoid arthritis cannot give of their best at school so their education suffers, as do their sports activities. Their social life is hampered, they cannot play with their friends, life becomes dull, boring and painful for them. Parents don't know what to do to rectify the situation so they call in the doctor. Blood tests and X-rays confirm that the child has rheumatoid arthritis. Bed rest in hospital may follow where the child may be given traction and drugs for arthritis, for example, Brufen, Indocid, or Feldene – there is quite an array of them. The drugs work for a little while and the patient is allowed to go home feeling better, but unfortunately the improvement is usually short lived. The effects of the drug wear off and the pain and stiffness return with full force. As drugs and pain can drain the body of iron, the patient may become anaemic. The doctor is called again, he or she increases the dosage of the drug or gives a stronger drug and the story repeats itself. The patient feels better for a little while and the same sorry saga starts all over again. How sad for the parents, they have to look on as their child cries with pain day and night, nobody gets any sleep, and the tension and frustration caused can lead to real problems in the family. Very often the child has gained so much weight as a side effect of the drugs or because of inactivity due to the pain of the illness, that it takes both parents to lift him or her out of bed and on to the toilet. Rheumatoid arthritis in a child is a very serious disease, because it frequently causes endocarditis (inflammation of the membrane lining the heart valves) which in many cases leads to permanent heart damage. One theory for the cause of rheumatic fever is that it is due primarily to infection by a streptococcus bacteria. In order for the streptococcus to produce the disease there must also be secondary causal factors. Enlarged tonsils and adenoids are important predisposing factors – constituting a path by which the infection can invade the system. Cold, wet, changes of temperature and fatigue may also act as predisposing factors. Sore throat, irregular joint pains, and slight malaise, may arise as preliminary symptoms, but as a rule the onset is abrupt and the disease is fully established within 24 hours. The joints are swollen and painful, the face is flushed, there are profuse sweats, the throat is often sore, the temperature high and the pain causes sleeplessness. The ordinary symptoms of fever are also marked: loss of appetite; thirst; constipation and highly coloured urine.

As a rule the large joints are involved. The knees, wrists, elbows and shoulder are red, hot and tender and extremely painful on movement. The inflammation wanders from joint to joint from day to day – one recovering as another is attacked. In uncomplicated cases, the acute symptoms subside within about ten days, but relapses are very common.

Involvement of the heart is more a part of the disease than a complication. Endocarditis is the most serious feature of acute rheumatic fever. It occurs in about 50% of cases and children rarely escape. The likelihood of endocarditis increases with the number of attacks of rheumatic fever. Myocarditis (inflammation of the heart muscle) nearly always accompanies endocarditis, and pericarditis (inflammation of the membrane surrounding the heart) if severe can lead to acute dilatation of the heart.

Skin complications are fairly common, blood spots in the skin may occur at the onset, especially in children. In convalescence tonics are necessary to combat the resulting anaemia and debility. Sufferers from rheumatic fever should subsequently take the greatest care to avoid damp, cold and chills. Of all the diseases that cast their shadow over childhood's happy hours rheumatoid arthritis is one of the worst.

Digestive troubles are common in children with rheumatic arthritis and many of them suffer with diarrhoea, mucous colitis or acidosis (a state in which abnormal acids appear in the child's urine). Since it is now widely accepted that arthritis is due to an excess of uric acid in the body, it is reasonable to assume that an attack of vomiting or diarrhoea could herald in an attack of arthritis.

Diet

To lessen the liability to billious attacks the child's diet should be well balanced, and should not contain an excess of starchy food. Sudden changes in diet, or even fright may bring on an attack of acidosis in some children. It is also essential that the diet should not be deficient in vitamins. Studies have shown that in animals lack or deficiency of Vitamins A or B lead to grave changes, such as atrophy, ulceration or colitis in the mucous lining of the intestine. As a result the animals waste, become anaemic and their temperature sinks. These symptoms are very similar to those found in children with rheumatoid arthritis. They too often suffer with anaemia, diarrhoea or colitis and a lower than normal temperature. It has also been found that if animals are deprived of Vitamins A and B the heart undergoes grave impairment. The cause of rheumatic heart disease is still unknown and it is possible that vitamin deficiency may play a part.

It is equally important that childrens' diets should not be deficient in mineral content. The fact that growing children need calcium needs no emphasis, but it is especially important for children who are prone to rheumatoid arthritis as it helps to diminish nervous irritability. Calcium and iodine metabolism are closely linked. Researchers have found that if a very small amount of iodine is added to the food of animals, it greatly increases their powers of absorbing and retaining calcium, phosphorus and nitrogen. We see then how important it is that childrens' diets should contain foodstuffs rich in both iodine and calcium.

For many years I have believed that arthritis is a deficiency disease. When a patient comes to my clinic for help, I immediately find out as far as possible which nutrients are lacking and supply them in the highest quality, together with an acid-free diet and an acid-removing treatment. It is my belief that a state of acidosis in my patient's body is brought about through a vitamin and mineral deficiency. The results I have obtained through nutritional therapy confirm my beliefs – the majority of my patients become well.

Prevention of this disease is most certainly better than cure, but before discussing methods of prevention it is necessary to emphasize that when a child develops symptoms of rheumatism, growing pains and the like we tend to think that it is a sudden illness – yesterday the child did not have rheumatism, but today he or she has. This is, however, not the case. Rheumatism, when it appears, is an end result, not a beginning. For years the child may have had deficiencies of vitamins, iodine and calcium, or may have had insufficient sunlight. Out of this badly nourished soul grows rheumatism, as diseases are the weeds that grow in human soil. If there is a history of rheumatism or arthritis in the child's family, then there is a real possibility that the child will inherit the same conditions, so efforts at prevention must begin at infancy.

Prevention

Some people seem to think that early diagnosis is the same as prevention, but this is not so. If rheumatism exists and can be diagnosed it has clearly not been prevented. If a child already has 'growing pains' it is a bit late to talk of prevention, especially when nearly 80% of children develop a rheumatic heart at the first attack of rheumatoid arthritis. It is quite clear then that our aim should be to prevent that first attack. We must begin from infancy upwards. It is in the pre-school years that parents should pay attention to the dangers associated with growing pains, sore throats, damp feet etc. Children with a family history of rheumatism can be the kind of children that tired mothers class as 'impossible' – very intelligent, highly emotional and excitable, but easily tired and prone to mope. However, a sulky child, in my opinion, is often just a tired child and should be soothed to rest, not chided into rebellion, tears and exhaustion. Even though they can be difficult and exasperating, I feel that children with a tendency to develop rheumatism are very often misunderstood.

These children are often restless and fidgety, they are prone to bouts of indigestion, diarrhoea or mucous colitis, and often develop skin rashes, for example, nettle rash or eczema.

Acute rheumatoid arthritis is strongly hereditary, so our responsibility lies in doing all we can to prevent children with the tendency towards the illness from developing it. The child's natural defences against weather changes may not be very good, so he or she should be allowed to adapt to them from infancy. These children should never be coddled as this could make them more sensitive. They must be in the open air as much as possible, and should wear light but warm clothing. They must never sit about in damp clothes or shoes. Cold dry air is very good for these children – it boosts up their metabolism and gives them a feeling of exhilaration. Air which is cold and damp is bad, and when out in these conditions they should be kept moving – not sitting around. They need all the sunshine they can get.

We must also endeavour to tone up their skin. Our weather is constantly changing from hot to cold, from dry to damp, we must train their skins to cope with these changes. Mothers should be taught that warm, cleansing baths should be followed by cold sponging or brisk friction with a coarse towel wrung out in cold water. In this way the child's nervous system and his or her skin are toned up.

Their mucous membranes too are very sensitive to weather changes. Damp houses favour rheumatism. If a house is damp the air feels cold and damp. If the windows in a damp house are closed and heat switched on the air gets warm, moist and stagnant. Breathing in this air day after day, a child can grow listless and suffer from loss of appetite. The mucous membrane of the throat can get dry making it very easy to catch a cold. Open window ventilation will ensure a constant supply of fresh air, and it is only in this way that a healthy condition of the mucous membrane can be maintained, and the liability to sore throats checked. Hygiene of the skin, mouth and teeth are also very important in the prevention of rheumatism.

The first symptoms of rheumatism usually occur in the muscles, and mothers should be warned of the gravity of 'growing pains'. It must be realized how closely the activity of the skin is bound up with muscle activity. When the muscles generate heat it is the skin's job to regulate that heat. To prevent rheumatism, the muscles, like the skin must be kept in a state of efficiency. Muscles need fuel, and they derive this fuel from the breaking down of starches, proteins, sugars and fats. Many children with a family history of rheumatism find it difficult to dispose of large amounts of these foodstuffs so their muscles get choked with waste products. Pain, stiffness and rheumatism are the outcome. The food intake and the muscle output must be well balanced. In other words children should be well fed, but not over fed. They should exercise but not over exercise. It should always be borne in mind that such children tire very quickly and recover slowly, they must never be allowed to get over fatigued and care should be taken that they get enough sleep. Mothers should be aware that young children require not only a long night's sleep but also a nap or two during the day. Rest is extremely important in the treatment of rheumatic heart disease, I feel very strongly that we should use rest as a means of preventing it.

When the child reaches school age everything possible should be done to make their school days pleasant. For the child who may be prone to rheumatism, health, not schooling should be the first priority. Anything that brings about mental or physical overstrain is unhelpful and the competitive side of work or play should be minimized.

The maintenance of good nutrition is extremely important. Routine weighing is also very important, sometimes it is the only means of detecting whether a child is thriving or not. If anaemia and weight loss are evident, the diet should be corrected and a good multivitamin which includes iron and Vitamin C given. Cantassium makes an excellent multivitamin for individual age ranges.

Control of the illness

We must now turn our thoughts to the presence of rheumatic symptoms – growing pains etc. All we can do once they are present is attempt to prevent their recurrence. Unfortunately rheumatism has a vicious tendency to recur again and again. So what can we do to prevent its recurrence? What I have suggested previously is applicable to the rheumatic child. Put your faith not in drugs but in the natural resources of the child's body. As I have said in my previous book: *Curing Arthritis – The Drug-Free Way*, the drugs for arthritis are the most dangerous drugs manufactured – they do not bring about a cure in any circumstances. These drugs produce many undesirable side effects, that once detected are irreversible. Many children have turned up at my clinic suffering from anaemia (drugs drain the body of iron), tinnitus (ringing noises in the ears), overweight, sleeplessness, irritability, nausea, ulceration, colitis, calcium deficiency, and zinc deficiency. Some drugs ruin the immune system rendering it totally incapable of fighting off infection. Arthritis drugs suppress pain and inflammation, but in the course of suppressing these symptoms conditions are set up in the body that predispose it to serious diseases, such as chronic bronchitis, pneumonia, cystitis, gall stones and a host of others.

Bed rest

When a child develops pain and stiffness he or she should be put to bed and the doctor called, never the reverse – the child should not be taken to the doctor. It should always be remembered that the heart may be involved and prompt rest may prevent the progress of heart trouble. A child with pain and stiffness should be in bed, because he or she may be suffering with heart disease – hence the danger of exertion. It is perhaps a good thing that the so-called growing pains, stiff neck and sore throats are painful, otherwise the doctor may not be called and the presence of a diseased heart could be overlooked. Children with rheumatism should be in bed: they need prolonged rest and careful treatment. They should be given an acid removing treatment of honey, cider vinegar and black molasses: 2 teaspoons honey dissolved in half a glass of warm water, to which is added 2 teaspoons cider vinegar. This drink is to be taken 3 times per day. It is very beneficial in dissolving the uric acids in the system. Additionally, ¼ teaspoon black molasses in a little hot water should be taken 3 times per day providing it does not cause diarrhoea.

Diet

Diet is very important, children should adopt an acid free diet avoiding: citrus fruits – oranges, lemons, grapefruits etc; fruit juices; tomatoes; tangerines; blackcurrants; redcurrants; plums, etc. Butter, cheese, fresh whole milk and cream must also be avoided. Low fat vegetable margarine, skimmed milk or dried milk are good substitutes. Cottage cheese may replace hard cheeses. Plenty of fish is permissible, as is lamb with the fat removed. No red meats are allowed. Plenty of green vegetables are highly recommended, as are nuts and seeds, except for salted peanuts. No crisps are allowed.

To compensate for the vitamins, minerals and protein lacking in the above diet, a range of these have been produced specially for my clinic. They include:

Protein – 1 heaped large teaspoonful daily
plus a range of vitamins and minerals

Vitamin C	250 mg	1 daily
B Complex	25 mg	1 daily
Calcium	300 mg	1 daily
Magnesium	39 mg	1 daily
Phosphorus	38 mg	1 daily
Vitamin E	200 IU	1 daily
Selenium	50 IU	1 daily
Iron	25 mg	1 daily
Kelp	250 mg	1 daily
Alfalfa	250 mg	1 daily
Vitamin A	2000 IU	1 daily
Vitamin D	200 IU	1 daily

For those who cannot take tablets the above has been condensed into a powder in capsule form, three to be taken per day for children over eight years old. The capsule can be broken and the powder taken in jam, porridge, soup or as preferred. Young children up to the age of eight require less. (*The above list is specially designed for children. The Margaret Hills Formula for adults is described in detail in Chapter 5.*)

As arthritis is a muscle wasting disease it is imperative that the patient receives a good quality protein to build up the muscles. I must now explain the reason for giving the recommended vitamins and minerals.

Vitamin B complex

Because of the pain experienced by arthritis sufferers and the frustration connected with the inactivity forced upon them, the nerves often become frayed. Nervous irritability is a very common symptom. This leads to headaches or migraines and very often to lack of sleep. The B Complex prescribed feeds those frayed nerves and enables the patient to become less irritable. In time the depression lifts and a feeling of calm is brought about that leads to sleepful, undisturbed nights. It is here that the healing begins.

Calcium, Magnesium and Phosphorus

Most patients suffer with very painful cramps due to lack of calcium salts in the tissues. To counteract this situation calcium, Magnesium and Phosphorus are given. When there is a lack of calcium there is a grave danger that the patient will develop a condition known as osteoporosis where the density of the bones is lost and they become brittle and break easily. Hair, teeth, nails and skin also suffer. Hair becomes dull, teeth decay, the skin becomes dry and the nails show ridges and break easily. Taking calcium, Magnesium and Phosphorus has a profound beneficial effect in these conditions.

Vitamin E and Selenium

Vitamin E and Selenium work together to increase circulation and strengthen the heart muscle. This is most important – as we have already discussed the heart invariably suffers when arthritis is present.

Iron and Vitamin C

Iron and Vitamin C work together. Most sufferers of arthritis are anaemic, therefore they need iron. Drugs drain the body of iron and the arthritis pain has the same effect. Vitamin C helps absorption of iron in the body, therefore iron should never be given without the accompanying Vitamin C, otherwise the iron can build up in the liver and cause liver poisoning. Also because of the withdrawal of citrus fruits from the diet it is very important that a vitamin C supplement is taken.

Kelp

Kelp is made from seaweed. It contains the minerals of the ocean and because arthritic patients are lacking in minerals I find this a very useful adjunct to the diet.

Alfalfa

Alfalfa has been noted recently to be very beneficial in the relief of arthritis. I have added this to my list of nutrients, knowing that it can do no harm and may do a lot of good.

The treatment described above of an acid removing treatment, accompanied by an acid-free diet supplemented with vitamins, minerals and protein is producing wonderful results in the relief of arthritis in young and old at my clinic in Coventry. Nothing happens overnight – no instant miracles – but a slow gradual return to health is invariably experienced.

It is very important that the stress factor is also reduced, as stress and tension have an adverse effect on the healing of arthritis. The stress factor will be discussed in Chapters 3 and 4, as I feel that it pertains more to the adult than to the child.

2

Arthritis in Adults

Statistics have shown that 95% of people in this country suffer with arthritis or rheumatism at some time in their lives. This really is a frightening situation, particularly when one considers that it is a preventable situation. To the nation, as to the individual, health and strength are the most precious possessions. A vast army of doctors, nurses, chemists and scientists of every kind are engaged in the struggle with disease. In my view, the medical army of every country is more expensive than its military force. Ill health is therefore a greater direct burden upon the nation than its security forces.

In my opinion, the occurrence of arthritis is the scourge of the nation today, and the invisible damage is very frequently vastly greater than the visible damage, even though the visible damage of arthritis is evident in a great many cases. As we go out to our daily work or shopping, we encounter so many people wearing surgical collars, callipers, built up shoes, leaning on walking sticks, frames or riding in invalid chairs. These are the visible signs, coupled, of course, with gross deformities of various parts of the body, particularly spine, hands and feet.

A great many people suffer with arthritis that is not so visible – they do not complain about actual arthritis necessitating professional advice – they are forever getting pains and aches and never, or rarely, feel up to the mark. A good healthy day is a rare occurrence.

People in perfect health can carry out their daily work without exertion or undue tiredness. They can perform intellectual work rapidly and excellently. A person with arthritis will find walking a mile or so exhausting, and moderate physical work beyond their strength, also exposure to change of temperature will make them ache all over. People with arthritis have no zest for work, they are crippled physically and mentally. Their work does not satisfy them nor the people for whom they work. Efficiency and good health go together as do inefficiency and reduced health.

Operating my clinic has brought home to me day after day how disastrous, to all, reduced health can be. Businessmen and managers become unable to make correct decisions, because their bad health prevents them seeing clearly. Millions of workers work slowly and inefficiently because their energy is low due to chronic ill health and physical discomfort.

Economic success in the modern world depends to a very large extent upon cooperation between employers and the employed. Social dissatisfaction and friction between employers and the employed have never been greater in this country than they are at present. At the same time we find that although people are now living longer, ill health and reduced health have never been more in evidence than they are today.

People become embittered through ill health and reduced health. Digestive troubles are responsible for depression, melancholy and despair in many many cases. A sound body and a sound mind go together, cheerfulness cannot be expected from those suffering from chronic arthritis. Health, happiness, prosperity and power go hand in hand. Ill health creates unhappiness, poverty and despair. The importance of the ill health factor upon the prosperity, happiness and greatness of nations cannot be over stated.

We are the only clinic in the country offering our type of treatment, and we are getting excellent results, so doctors are now beginning to refer patients to us, the word is spreading and we are inundated with enquiries and people wanting to attend. Obviously, we can only do so much so we have to keep the number of appointments under control. Most people can carry out their treatment at home, and with this in mind we have developed a system of treatment by post that is working very well, and we now treat patients in many parts of the world.

However, we always make an effort to give an appointment to children, young adults and people who are suffering severe side effects of drugs. We help them to get off the drugs and in doing this both their mental and physical health improves.

Adults of 18–30 years old with arthritis

Adult patients afflicted with either rheumatoid or osteoarthritis whose ages range from 18 years to 30 years, will usually be offered an appointment when they call the clinic, as we realize that these people are starting out in life and need our expert and immediate attention. Most of these people are on a string of dangerous drugs and many of them are suffering from side effects. All arthritics suffer in the same sort of way to a greater or lesser degree. The same standard treatment applies to everybody, but some people are so low and their immune system so under-nourished, they need a lot more than the standard treatment. Drugs for arthritis drain the body of so many nutrients, such as iron, that most of my patients are anaemic. Many suffer with osteo-porosis (brittle bones) caused by a lack of calcium, and many have wasting and weakness of the muscles. All these conditions must be corrected and this doesn't happen overnight. With some it is a long trek back along the road to recovery.

Those who have not been on drugs for arthritis see results much sooner. It is a constant source of worry to me that steroid drugs are so widely used, because they have a very severe side effect of causing muscle weakness, thus adding to the muscle weakness already associated with arthritis. I see some patients in the 18 to 30 age group who can scarcely move a muscle – the strength is not there, and the condition is made worse by taking steroids. Isn't it time the doctors looked into an alternative to drugs? The fears and frustrations of the young people I see are devastating. Some are doing A levels, some are at university and some in their first jobs. They come for an appointment scarcely able to walk – many of them put on an enormous amount of weight due to the steroids they have been prescribed, and on examination of urine samples, invariably I find blood and protein present due to steroids. Very often we find a rise in blood pressure – this too can be due to the drugs. These young people start to relate their history of arthritis – the blood tests, the X-rays, the drugs, the doctor's words: 'learn to live with it', and then they burst into tears.

If the doctors who utter those words had ever experienced the pain of arthritis they would realize the death sentence they were passing on these young people. I know it is very frustrating for doctors – they realize that their only treatment for arthritis is drugs, they also know the drugs won't cure anything and that they only add to the misery with their side effects. It was most encouraging, some time ago, when a patient related to me that her consultant had said he was delighted that she was partaking of my treatment instead of his 'poison'.

Infections and antibiotics in arthritis

Inflammation of the throat is commonly associated with exposure to cold in arthritic, rheumatic and gouty conditions. It reveals itself by heat and dryness in the throat, with soreness on swallowing. There is slight fever, and an aching back and limbs are commonly present. As a result, when this happens, the doctor is called and he prescribes an antibiotic. This aggravates arthritis and the unfortunate patient suffers an upsurge of pain. Usually antibiotics are administered alone, rather than alongside Vitamin B complex. This practice can lead to the patient developing thrush – *Candida albicans*, a most uncomfortable condition that is very hard to get rid of. When I was a young nurse in hospital, forty three years ago, it was a recognized thing that all patients taking antibiotics were given Vitamin B complex as a matter of course. I did not realize then the full value of this practice, but today it is brought home to me time after time why this happened. Antibiotic literally means 'anti-life'. In many cases antibiotics can kill off the germ that is causing the sore throat or whatever, and in that way they are good, but they can also kill off the much needed friendly bacteria that inhabit the whole mucous system of the body. This can leave the patient with no defences and an extensive growth of the yeast-like fungus *Candida albicans*, is the result. If a high dosage of Vitamin B Complex is administered with the antibiotic this situation does not occur.

Candida albicans

Candida albicans is a form of thrush affecting the whole mucous membrane from mouth to anus. White patches of a yeast-like fungus appear on the tongue, palate or cheek, these spread extensively to the pharynx, oesophagus, the intestine, in fact the complete digestive system is affected. The infection renders the patient reluctant to eat, leading to a deficiency of much needed nutrients. The discomfort of the mouth ulcers and anal itching also caused by the infection can be quite unbearable. Treatment of *Candida albicans* varies with its severity.

Treatment of mild or one-off attacks

If the condition is mild or a one-off attack, then the following treatment is effective: a good diet in conjunction with a good multivitamin (Cantamega 2000 is the best in my opinion) taken once a day; plus Vitamin B complex (100 mg daily) to nourish the intestinal flora; and 1000 mg of Vitamin C daily to cleanse the blood. An oral supplement of *Lactobacillus acidophilus* (in the form of a dry culture – 1 teaspoon, three times per day), should also be taken to reinoculate the bowel with helpful bacteria. This treatment programme has been extremely successful in reducing *Candida albicans* infections.

Chronic Candida albicans

Typically a chronic candida sufferer is female. She comes for an appointment to my clinic in desperation. She has been to her doctor who, having listened to all her symptoms, has come to the conclusion that it is her age and that she is suffering from neurosis. She has been for various alternative treatments, for example, acupuncture but nothing has worked. She knows she is not neurotic but she also knows that her symptoms are very real and uncomfortable.

After spending a lot of time questioning my patient about her past health history, I invariably find that at some time she has had to have a series of antibiotics for bronchitis, cystitis, or some other condition. She thinks that the trouble must stem from then as she hasn't been 'right' since. I then ask her to explain her symptoms – they seem endless. Her depression is awful, she bursts into tears at the drop of a hat – no wonder her doctor thought it was nerves. She feels so tired that she doesn't want to do anything, and she has no interest in anything. She also has uncomfortable, embarrassing itching of her vagina and her abdomen is swollen. She feels bloated, and very often she gets diarrhoea. She gets frequent attacks of cystitis, and this is why she has had to take so many antibiotics. She also had mouth ulcers, and gets a lot of embarrassing wind and belching. On top of all this she thinks she may have arthritis because she gets a lot of aching in her muscles, tingling, numbness and swelling in her joints, headaches, spots before her eyes, and she loses her balance sometimes. Also her mouth is dry and her breath is bad.

From the description of her symptoms I realize straight away that she is a chronic candida sufferer. All the above symptoms and many more are connected with this condition. What a relief it is to this lady that at last somebody has put a name to her suffering. However, naming the condition is one thing but curing it is another, and this is no easy task for my patient. As I have already explained, the condition has arisen as a result of antibiotic treatment without Vitamin B complex. Of course common foods we eat that, unknown to us, contain hormones and antibiotics also contribute. Sometimes it can take months to correct the damage that has occurred. For example, the long term infection may have caused an imbalance in the intestine, leaving the digestive system unable to digest certain foods. Toxic wastes are then produced, which manifest as skin complaints, digestive disorders, infections and unaccountable aches and pains. The immune system has become so depleted that it is unable to resist viruses and bacteria.

Treatment of chronic Candida albicans

The treatment of such cases consists of a diet specially formulated to starve the offending bacteria in the digestive tract, and to promote the health of the friendly bacteria.

The foods that may be eaten are as follows: vegetables, especially cooked broccoli, cauliflower, swede and vegetables of the cabbage family; meat and chicken that are unsmoked and antibiotic and steroid-free; unsmoked fish; game meat; shell fish; and eggs.

Safflower oil 4–6 teaspoons daily, linseed oil 1–3 teaspoons daily, plenty of filtered water and mineral water, fresh vegetable juices, and psyllium husks for fibre may also be taken. Also eat as much garlic as you can to clean the blood. It has been found that linseed oil is an excellent source of linolenic acid which will break down fats and cholesterol thus ridding the intestines of a lot of gluten. Avoid all other foods until you feel better and then start to reintroduce them one at a time, looking out for a recurrence of symptoms. If any symptoms do recur you must discontinue that particular food.

It was originally thought that yoghurt was good for candida patients because it does help to normalize the intestinal flora. Lately, however, it has been found that the large amount of milk in yoghurt feeds the fungus so it is best to steer clear of yoghurt. In conjunction with the above diet the taking of Superdophilus (a Lactobacillus Acidophilus powder formulated to produce a potent, natural antibiotic) is most important to restore the flora in the intestinal system.

The foods not allowed are as follows: fruit of any sort; fruit juices (these can be introduced as symptoms subside); yoghurt; mushrooms; dried fruits; and nuts and seeds. Also not allowed are: all sugars; honey; sweeteners; fructose; glucose; malt; syrups; any foods containing yeast (for example bread and yeast spreads); dairy products (milk, cheese, butter, etc.); fermented foods (for example, soya sauce and beer); smoked meats and smoked fish; monosodium glutamate; peanuts; pistachios; alcoholic beverages; birth control pills; preservative; and frozen peas.

Following the above programme helps boost the immune system and enables it to do its job of protecting the body. Vitamin supplementation is very necessary while following the programme, but beware of cheaper vitamins as these can do more harm than good: a lot of them are yeast-based, supplying yeast to a body that is already over populated with a yeast fungi.

I can think of no better vitamin supplementation than that described in Chapter 1, page 10. An adult needs double the strength, in conjunction with the following: L-arginine (an amino acid known to boost the immune system) 4×500 mg tablets per day for the first six weeks. Aloe vera reduces inflammation and can also be a great help in this condition.

Results can be very slow to manifest but, like chronic arthritis *Candida albicans* is a long standing condition and one cannot expect instant results. However, with patience and perseverance results do come, and they are well worth waiting and striving for.

It is very disconcerting to realize that taking antibiotics without Vitamin B complex can have such far reaching, long, and devastating effects on the human body, and what a dreadful thought that the unfortunate arthritis sufferer now has two chronic diseases to cope with instead of one.

Doctors usually give Nystatin to cure *Candida albicans* infection. This antibiotic does kill the parasitic yeast but it also produces side effects such as nausea, stomach pains and depression. Killing the offending yeast parasite is, unfortunately, only half the story, and antibiotics do not nourish the friendly intestinal flora. In fact they can destroy it, meaning that a return of the condition is inevitable. The treatment combining

Superdophilus and diet takes longer to have its effect, but when it does results are complete and long lasting with no side effects. Patients end up with a thoroughly cleansed body and a strengthened immune system, and a feeling of well-being they have not experienced for years. Fortunately, relatively few 18–30 year olds develop chronic candida infection. As a rule they don't need a lot of antibiotics, but we do get the odd one coming to the clinic who through recurrent bronchitis, sore throat or whatever had to take a series of antibiotics and has a long-term infection.

Most young adults get very quick results on the diet and treatment we prescribe for them. For example a 14 year old girl from Ireland, who had attended every consultant her parents could think of only to be told nothing could be done, spent six months on the Margaret Hills Treatment and reported that all cramps, pins and needles and sleeplessness had disappeared. Her father said they now 'had to put the brakes on' as she looked so well, positive and happy. After just six months she had cut out her drugs completely and was getting very little pain.

Chronic osteoarthritis

An example of someone suffering from chronic arthritis is the woman whose husband brings her for an appointment to the clinic. I take note as he opens the car door for her and proceeds to lift her out, first her legs and then her body. I can see her weight is quite a strain on him, and the look of agony on her face because of the movement has to be seen to be believed. He hands her her walking frame or sticks, or if she can't walk at all he brings the wheelchair. I sit her down in the clinic, her husband takes a chair beside her, and I take her case history whilst my assistant examines her urine and takes her blood pressure.

They tell me that they have come to the clinic because for years the woman has been attending hospital and taking all sorts of drugs, that have worked for a little while, but now are doing no good at all. She is now on a high dosage of steroids but is getting worse, and the consultant has said he can do no more for her. I ask her how she came to know of the clinic. She says that a neighbour or friend has been for treatment and got wonderful results, and that if she could just get a little relief from her pains, she would be very grateful.

As I proceed with the consultation I observe the anaemic look on her face – drugs and pain drain the body of iron. I ask her when she last had a blood test. She says six months ago and that she was anaemic then, but also that she has been anaemic for years and has been taking Ferrograd (an iron tablet) for years. Her hair is dull and lifeless, her skin is pale and her eyes lack any lustre. It is obvious that she lacks calcium – the ridges on her nails are pronounced and the rough skin on her hands all tell the same story. When there is a lack of calcium the skin, hair, teeth, bones and nails all suffer. I look at her nails and she tells me that they break very easily: lack of calcium is again to blame. Her nails also have a scattering of white spots which she says she has had for years. I tell her that these spots show that her immune system is very undernourished through a lack of zinc, and that this can be due to drug therapy. Steroids suppress the immune system and drain the body of many nutrients. Her skin is paper thin and her legs are ulcerated – all this can be a direct result of taking steroids. The disadvantages of taking steroids, in my opinion, far outweigh the advantages. The dangerous side effects of steroids are numerous and include the following: high blood pressure; sodium and water retention; potassium loss; and muscle weakness. Bearing in mind that arthritis is a muscle wasting disease, and that steroids also cause muscle weakness, it is no wonder that the arthritis sufferers often feel so drained of strength that they can't even lift a cup. Steroids can also cause diabetes and osteoporosis, which is a great danger especially in older people as it may cause vertebral collapse. Mental disturbances may occur, and a serious paranoid state or depression with risk of suicide may be induced, particularly in patients with a history of mental disorder. Peptic ulceration is a recognized complication which may result in haemorrhage or perforation of the stomach or duodenum. Suppression of symptoms may allow septicaemia or tuberculosis to reach an advanced stage before being recognized. High doses of steroids can cause Cushing's syndrome with moon face, purple striae over the abdomen, and acne. The administration of steroids suppresses the adrenal glands in the body and may lead to atrophy (wasting) – this can persist for years after the steroids have been stopped. Steroids give a feeling of well being which is quite unnatural. Steroids should not be used unless the benefits justify the hazards, as the complications and side effects of the therapy can be far more serious than the disease itself. Bearing in mind this list of side effects it is no wonder that so many devastated arthritis sufferers want to find a way of discontinuing their steroids. Some of my patients develop a lot of symptoms, and are willing to do anything to discontinue their drugs. With some people this takes a long time, depending on the length of time they have been taking steroids and on the dosage. Some patients are on nonsteroid drugs as well as steroids. This complicates things too – normally we get them to discontinue the nonsteroid drugs first and then very gradually start to reduce the steroids.

Nonsteroid drugs should be taken with great caution as ulceration and allergic disorders can occur. They should not be given to people with peptic ulcers and they should only be given to older people as a last resort, and then only in very low dosage. The side effects are numerous – gastrointestinal discomfort is a common symptom and nausea, diarrhoea and, occasionally, bleeding also occur. Angioneurotic oedema, asthma, rashes, headache, dizziness, vertigo and hearing disturbances such as tinnitus can also occur. As can blood disorders and fluid retention. Nonsteroid drugs should not be given to anybody with a kidney problem, and they should always be taken after food. Aspirin too, if taken in large doses can produce tinnitus, dizziness, deafness, and in fact many of the same side effects as the other nonsteroid drugs.

Of patients suffering with arthritis, 99% are on one drug or another and unfortunately the vast majority are suffering from one or more severe side effects. Some of my patients say the ringing noises in their ears are driving them mad, and a lot of them describe the arthritis in the head as 'creepy crawlies'. No matter how they try to relieve these conditions, they can't, they are with them day and night. With most people the 'creepy crawly' effect subsides as the arthritis subsides. This leads me to believe that the condition is associated with a trapped nerve in the cervical vertebrae due to acid deposits. However, the ringing noises usually stay, even when the drug is discontinued.

This then is the story of someone suffering from chronic rheumatoid or osteoarthritis. She has come to see me because she is frightened of the side effects of her drugs. She wants to discontinue them, and will do anything to achieve this. In the following chapters I will relate various case histories of young and old, and results obtained on treatment through my clinic.

3

A Selection of Case Histories

This Chapter contains a selection of Case Histories taken from my notes. I am sure a lot of arthritis sufferers will be able to identify with them, and derive the courage and perseverence needed to continue with their treatment even when they seem to have come to a standstill.

As the number of patients wanting an appointment at my clinic is far beyond its capacity – there are not enough hours in the day in which to see them all – we have devised a questionnaire (see page 25) that we send out to all enquirers. Prospective patients fill in and return the questionnaire. The information we receive tells us the age and sex of the patient and whether the patient is taking steroids, and/or, other drugs for arthritis. We ask if they suffer from nerves, heart trouble, diabetes, headaches, migraine, loss of sleep, cramp, pins and needles, pain, excessive tiredness, or depression. We also ask if they have ridges on their nails, if their nails contain white spots, and whether they are under or overweight. We also need to know if they are taking any other drugs and what these drugs are for. We also find out for how long they've had arthritis, whether they have any other illnesses and whether there are other comments they would like to make.

All this information has a direct bearing on the treatment. We make a point of seeing all children at the clinic before we start treatment, also all young people, and anybody we feel may need our help in discontinuing their drugs. Some people are on very strong steroids and suffering from side effects, for example overweight, high blood pressure, blood and protein in their urine, or anaemia. These people come back time and time again until they have discontinued their drugs, and the side effects have been dealt with naturally.

Some people have been patients here for 2½ years, we get to know them very well, and take a personal interest in them. They look forward to their appointments and are delighted to be able to tell us the positive results they have noticed from day to day, like being able to lift their arms to do their hair – perhaps something

MARGARET HILLS CLINIC – QUESTIONNAIRE

To obtain this questionnaire and supportive literature, please send a stamped, self-addressed envelope to the clinic. When you have completed it, please return it to the clinic.

NAME .... (PLEASE PRINT)

ADDRESS ....

....

Post Code ....

Age .... Male/Female Tel No ....

Are you diabetic?

Can you get into the bath?

Do you suffer from the following:

Nerves?	Pins and needles?
Heart trouble?	Pain?
Headaches?	Excessive tiredness?
Migraine?	Depression?
Loss of sleep?	Nails with ridges?
Cramp?	Nails with white spots?

Describe your weight: OVER/UNDER/AVERAGE

Details of any drugs you are taking:

Name of drug	Prescribed for	Dosage	How long taken for

How long have you had arthritis?

Details of any other illnesses ....

....

Any other comments ....

....

they haven't been able to do this for years. It brings home to me how much we healthy ones take for granted, I thank God for my own good health and that of my family, and I also thank Him for the improvement in my patients' health.

Case History 1 – Mrs K

On the 25th May 1987 Mrs K wrote the following letter to the clinic:

Dear Mrs Hills,
Thank you so very much for your book *'Curing Arthritis – The Drug-Free Way'*. It read like a revelation to me – I couldn't believe it because all the doctors had said is that there is nothing that can be done.

I have been following the advice in your book for three weeks and I have definitely improved. The pains in my neck and shoulder are much easier, although to my surprise, because I have been eating very well, I have lost a little weight. I have known I had arthritis of the spine for about 5 years. I have tried not to take the drugs, but sometimes I have to. That was before I started your diet – I have not taken a tablet since. I am fifty-one years of age, I thank you most sincerely for your wonderful book and for your wonderful courage, I would be grateful if you would send me the latest details on your treatment. With all God's blessing to you – Yours in Jesus – Mrs K.

We sent her a questionnaire which she filled in and returned on June 10th 1987. On processing the questionnaire we learned that Mrs K was 51 years old and suffering from her nerves, she suffered migraine headaches, lost sleep, had a lot of pain, felt very tired, and was overweight. She had been taking Prempak C for the menopause and Temazepam for sleeplessness, although she had now discontinued these. She took Migraleve for headaches and Fenbid for arthritis. She had had arthritis for 5 years.

Before filling in our questionnaire she had gone along to the health food shop and bought honey, cider vinegar and black molasses, and having taken these products, in conjunction with

Vitamin B6, she reported in her questionnaire that her migraine was much better. She also said that since taking Vitamin B complex her sleeping was much better. She had no other illness. She had also discontinued her Fenbid.

On June 15th we replied to her questionnaire:

Dear Mrs K,

You may continue to take your Prempak C for the time being although when on our treatment your menopausal symptoms should subside appreciably. Also, as you go through this treatment you should not need your Temazepam, or Migraleve as the sleeplessness and migraine are connected with your arthritis. As that condition disperses in your body, the sleeplessness and migraine should be relieved and hopefully overcome. Please do not resort to taking Fenbid. When in pain, 2 paracetamol should suffice.

In addition to the Margaret Hills Formula nutrition enclosed, you need to take an instant protein nutritional drink once daily in place of a meal – preferably breakfast. Please let us know how you are getting on as you reorder.

On June 30th we received a reorder from Mrs K with a little note to tell us that she had read 'Curing Arthritis – The Drug-Free Way' in April, and had started the diet prescribed, and since starting on that diet she had felt a lot better. She said the interval between the pains was much longer and when the pain came it was less acute. She had lost half a stone since April 30th, and she felt very well. She said she had much less migraine, in fact she had only had three bouts since April 30th and they were not as acute as usual. She was also sleeping much better.

On July 28th another reorder arrived from Mrs K, again with a little note. In her own words: 'The pain is now an ache! I am still 10½ stone and very pleased about that. I feel very well'. She wished to know if cherries, grapes or quinces, grape juice, black cherries and peanut butter are permissable in the diet. She thanked us for all our help and said she was telling many people about our treatment.

We sent off her order and answered her queries:

Dear Mrs K,
We are so pleased that you are getting on well. Sorry, cherries, grapes and quinces are not permitted – they are too acid, as are grape juice and black cherries – you may have a little peanut butter, and you will find apricot diabetic jam is delicious. Very best wishes.

On September 1st we received another order with the following note:

Thank you, all is well, I've had odd days with quite a bit of pain but not acute. I am quite free of pain most of the time. I am going to Italy for a week on September 19th, I will take the honey, cider vinegar and black molasses with me. Apart from that I will try to keep to the diet and vitamins, but as we are going to a hotel with breakfast and evening meal I may find it difficult – much love.

At this stage we felt we had gained our patient's confidence. The ending of her note with 'much love' was very encouraging and here started a lovely friendship which was to last right through to June 7th 1988, when she informed us that she was totally clear of arthritis.

However, in the meantime, she had various flare-ups. These flare-ups (bouts of pain and stiffness) are an attempt by the body to rid itself of the arthritis, and are very essential. They are uncomfortable while they last, but if not treated with a suppressive drug, and encouraged to come out naturally with the aid of bathing in epsom salts, massage with olbas oil and rest, the patient experiences a tremendous feeling of well being and sense of achievement, and is thrilled to have mastered the pain without drugs. Mrs K was no exception. On November 16th 1987 we received a further note saying:

Dear Margaret,
Thank you for your help so far. I am still improving though slowly. I still have a great deal of discomfort in my neck, but no acute pain. My feet are very much better, I can walk without arch supports, I do get occasional pain. Could you

please tell me if yellow tomatoes are acid free? All best wishes.

It is very comforting to patients to realize that they can have a constant rapport with the Clinic, either by phone or letter. There is always somebody there to encourage, sympathize or give advice. I feel very lucky to have my daughter Christine working in the clinic with me. Christine has been involved since I started, and is very dedicated to the work, nothing is too much trouble. She will do anything to comfort the patient and ease the suffering.

Our reply to Mrs K's note on November 24th went as follows:

Dear Mrs K,
I am so pleased that you are still improving. Just keep on keeping on! In my opinion all tomatoes have got acid in them, best to steer clear. Have a lovely Christmas and our very best wishes to you.

Christmas passed and January 21st brought another letter from Mrs K which read:

Dear Margaret,
Thank you for all your help so far. I must say the condition in my neck is stable. I don't have much pain. I can still feel a stiffness but most of the time I don't notice it. I can walk now, I don't wear arch supports and can wear any suitable shoe. Do you think this would be a good time to review the situation and lessen the taking of the treatment? Please tell me how to continue.

We replied to Mrs K:

Dear Mrs K,
We are very sorry but we cannot reduce your nutrition as yet. We have found that many people who have reduced their nutrition too soon have had a return of arthritis, and have had to restart the full treatment again. This situation we do not want to occur and we are very sure that you don't want this either. Even though it may mean carrying on for a few more

months, it will be well worth the effort. When you have been clear of arthritis for three months – that means no arthritic pain or swelling, we can then discontinue your protein and reduce your nutrition. Our very best wishes to you.

Mrs K carried on with her treatment as advised until June 7th when the following little note arrived:

Dear Margaret,
Thank you so much for all your help. I am most grateful. I have no pain and am very well. I would like to know how to continue. Yours sincerely.

Our reply on June 14th went as follows:

Dear Mrs K,
We are so pleased that you are now free of arthritis, and hopefully the return of those painful symptoms will not occur. However, it is very necessary to take a Margaret Hills Formula sachet every other day plus one Vitamin C tablet on the days you do not take the formula. This means you will be sending in for one box of Formula and one packet of Vitamin C every other month. It is very necessary to continue in this way for the duration of your life so that the acids will be kept down in your body, thus preventing a return of the arthritis. You may now discontinue your protein powder. Eat plenty of fish, chicken, cottage cheese etc. Take a cider vinegar drink once daily, and hopefully good health will be yours from now on. Our very best wishes to you.

That letter was sent on June 14th 1988. Since then Mrs K has been in very good health. She is well, happy and free of all signs of arthritis as she tells us in her letter written November 28th 1989:

Dear Margaret Hills,
I am now very well indeed, I have no stiffness and no pain, I am so grateful. I have sold many of your books and now keep three at home all the time to give or sell to those who need them. I still keep to the diet, though not so strictly as I did

before. Now, I do not take the black molasses, I still have two glasses of honey and cider vinegar daily, usually warm. It's a delightful drink and I know it will keep the acids down, I think I shall always keep this up. I still keep to lamb, chicken, fish and find many different ways to serve these, no feelings of being deprived. Also, I keep to food free of animal fat – no citrus fruits at all. Of course salads and vegetables are very much part of the diet and cottage cheese.

I keep very well indeed, I do not have migraines now – these were very bad before I started on your treatment, but I've hardly had one since. I sleep well and have lots of energy. My feet were very bad but I can now walk faster than my husband. Also my neck, I found it hard to do my desk work, or reverse the car – no problem now. I thank you very much indeed once again. I do hope many more people find out about your treatment – with best wishes for your new book and all you do.

I have never met Mrs K, but I feel so honoured and so humble that through me she has been able to lead a normal life and be free of pain. She is one of thousands who have benefited from advice and treatment sought from this clinic.

Being informed and taking responsibility for one's illness is very necessary to help ensure that one is getting the best treatment available. It is brought home to me day after day that steroid and nonsteroid drugs are not a good treatment for arthritis because of their terrible side effects.

I call the treatment I give for arthritis 'complementary' not 'alternative' because often I have to ask a patient to go back onto a particular drug, because of the pain involved if the drug is withdrawn too quickly. Also, of course, many patients are taking other drugs for various diseases, such as heart, thyroid and blood pressure problems. It is very important that doctors' treatments for these conditions are adhered to. It is also very important that my patients realize that my sole aim is to make them feel better, whether this is through my therapy alone or a combination of my treatment and the doctor's.

Case History 2 – Mrs G

Mrs G enquired about our treatment on November 7th 1986. We

sent her the usual questionnaire which she filled in and returned to us. Having processed it we decided she did not need an appointment at the clinic. She could quite easily carry out the treatment at home. She had been diagnosed with arthritis about 3 weeks previously. She suffered from very occasional migraine, occasional cramp and pins and needles and twinges of pain. She was of average weight for her height and she had no other illness. She informed us that 3 weeks previously she had had quite a severe pain in one knee which had thrown her off balance. Since then it had improved, but she wondered if it was possible to have treatment more 'as a preventive measure' and she did not want to start taking drugs. She said she had read my book '*Curing Arthritis – The Drug-Free Way*' and my approach to the disease appealed to her. She was 61 years of age.

We sent Mrs G our standard treatment consisting of Margaret Hills Formula and Protein, with a comprehensive diet programme and advice on taking cider vinegar, honey and black molasses. We also explained the benefit of taking epsom salts baths.

She carried out the treatment as advised, sending in for her monthly supplies.

On February 25th 1987 we received a little note to say: 'The arthritis in my knee seems to have gone and I have had no twinges for about a fortnight. I understand I should continue with the treatment for another three months'. She sent us a cheque for her usual monthly supply and ended her note: 'With grateful thanks for your help and advice'. On October 23rd 1987 she sent us a little note saying she was feeling extremely well, and that she had no more aches in her knee. On February 22nd she telephoned to say she had now been free from pain for over three months and that she needed our advice on how to carry on in future.

We advised her, as we advised all our other patients who achieve that happy state, as follows: To take one sachet of Margaret Hills Formula every other day, plus one Vitamin C tablet on the day the sachet is not taken, the reason for this being that Margaret Hills Formula contains 500 mg Vitamin C. Therefore Vitamin C, which is very necessary in the daily diet, is not missed. We also told her she may now discontinue her protein, but that she must make sure that she has a good wholefood, protein-filled nourishing diet, avoiding as much as possible the offending acids. One daily dose of cider vinegar and honey was also recommended to keep the acids down. We congratulated her and wished her good luck.

In February 1989 she wrote to us as follows: 'The success of the Margaret Hills Formula against arthritis and rheumatism was proved to me when I visited my optician. About two years ago I went to him to renew my spectacles. He looked at the old pair I was using and asked: "Have you got rheumatism?" I replied: "It's funny you should say that, because my right knee is very painful and now the left one has started to be painful also." '

'Shortly after this visit I started taking the Margaret Hills Formula and protein with the diet, with excellent results. When the time came to return to my optician he again looked at the frames and said: "You no longer have rheumatism". My reply was: "No I don't, how did you know that?" He answered that on the previous frames the gold under the earpieces was very discoloured due to the acid on the skin working its way under the plastic coverings for the ears, and causing the metal to become stained. The new frames I had been using while I was taking your treatment were not marked at all. I also had no more pain.' She ended her letter by saying: 'If this testimony is any use to you please use it. With my very grateful thanks.' Mrs G is still totally clear of arthritis.

The story of Mrs G goes to show that the sooner the correct treatment for rheumatism or arthritis is adopted, the sooner the disease is brought under control, and the less suffering is experienced. It did not take Mrs G very long to rid herself of the uric acids that were causing her pain, and now all she has to do is carry on with the advice given to her. If she has a problem she knows she can contact the clinic either by phone or letter – she will be helped whenever possible.

Case History 3 – Mrs W

The story of Mrs W is different. Mrs W is a 68-year-old lady suffering with high blood pressure, who contacted us in early August 1988. She had had a heart bypass operation in December 1985. Her circulation was very poor, she was taking a quarter of a soluble aspirin tablet each day for this. Her doctor had prescribed Kalten for her high blood pressure. She was getting severe headaches, cramp and a lot of pain in her neck, shoulders and the base of her spine. She was getting very little sleep. She had suffered with angina for 6 years and had had arthritis for 8–9 years. Her nails were very ridged.

Having processed her questionnaire we decided she did not need a clinic appointment. She could carry out our treatment at home, in conjunction with her doctor's treatment for high blood pressure and poor circulation. On August 26th we wrote to her as follows:

Dear Mrs W,
Please continue to take your Kalten and aspirin until your doctor says otherwise. Because of your many and varied symptoms we must suggest that you take a course of Zinc for three months in conjunction with the Margaret Hills Formula and Protein. Our very best wishes to you. Please let us know how you get on as you reorder.

In Chapter 4 I shall enlarge on the value of taking Zinc and why we ask most of our patients to take it.

On October 3rd the following letter arrived from Mrs W:

Dear Mrs Hills,
I have been taking your formula for just a few days and now I have started to have a touch of diarrhoea and nausea. I have ordered the Zinc tablets but have not received them as yet. I have discontinued the treatment for the present as I am going on holiday from October 10th–15th and do not wish to feel ill while I am away. I would appreciate your advice as soon as possible.

Our reply to Mrs W went like this:

Dear Mrs W,
On no account should you have discontinued taking your Formula and Protein – the diarrhoea had nothing to do with that, but you may have been taking too much molasses, even though it says on your diet sheet to start with half a teaspoonful and build up gradually. On the other hand it is

quite possible that you may have caught a bug – there have been a lot about causing diarrhoea and nausea. Hopefully you have now restarted your treatment and will continue according to our instructions.

Mrs W had restarted the treatment and continued with it. She sent us a letter on December 2nd which went like this:

Dear Mrs Hills,
Just to inform you how I am going on with the treatment. My weight is constant. I am still having pain, but I am getting a day free from pain occasionally, which I was not getting before. I am sending in for my third month's supply of Zinc tablets which you advised at the beginning of my treatment. I should like to know if I have to carry on with these. Yours sincerely.

We advised Mrs W to now discontinue her Zinc but to carry on taking her Formula and protein also paying attention to her diet, epsom salts baths, etc.
   This she continued to do and on June 27th 1989 she wrote the following note:

Dear Mrs Hills,
Just to let you know that my arthritis is clearing up very well, and I think I shall soon be free of it. She also said that she was getting a sickly feeling and wondered if it was the treatment she was having from us.

On July 3rd we replied thanking her for her letter and telling her that we were pleased that she was improving, also reassuring her that nothing in our treatment could make her feel sickly. We advised her to have a word with her doctor if the condition persisted and to let us know his comments.
   The condition must have cleared up because we heard no more from Mrs W until September 20th when she wrote the following note:

Dear Mrs Hills,
I am writing to let you know that I now feel my arthritis has cleared up. I am extremely grateful for your help – it feels

grand to be free of pain after so many years. I saw the doctor about my sickness and he gave me antacid tablets.

We replied in the following manner:

Dear Mrs W,
Thank you for your letter. We are so pleased that you are now free of pain, but we do not wish you to discontinue this treatment until you have been without any signs of arthritis for a clear three months. In our experience, people who discontinue the treatment too soon frequently experience a return of their former symptoms. We know that you would not wish this and feel that another three months to make completely sure that your body is free of all acids would be a period well spent. You have now been on this treatment for twelve months and when you started you had arthritis in your neck, shoulders and base of your spine. You also suffered with headaches, sleeplessness, cramp and a great deal of pain. You have done very well over the twelve month period to become free of all those symptoms, so please do not leave this treatment off too soon. With very best wishes.

Mrs W took our advice and on December 4th 1989 she wrote again telling us that she is still free from pain and all symptoms of arthritis, and reminding us that her extended three months were now up. She thanked us once again for our help and she wished to know how to carry on in the future. We were delighted and replied as follows:

Dear Mrs W,
You have been very patient in following our instructions and we are so pleased that you are now free from pain – this is a great achievement. Continue to take your Margaret Hills Formula nutrition – one sachet every two days – and in addition to this 500 mg Vitamin C every other day, i.e. on the days you do not take the sachet.
You may now discontinue your protein supplement, if you wish, also the epsom salts baths and the molasses, but make sure that you have a good wholefood, protein-filled nourishing diet, avoiding the offending acids. Take one daily dose of

cider vinegar and honey. We enclose a revised reorder form to help you to order the correct items in future. Many congratulations and very good luck for the future.

On January 1st 1990 Mrs W wrote again saying that her arthritis had started in the mid-seventies, and added: 'For many years I was taking painkillers and massaging with different oils, but to no avail. I was in constant pain in my neck and back. In the autumn of 1988 I read an article in my local paper about how you had suffered and cured yourself with your formula, protein and diet, so I decided to give it a try. I am so glad to say that in fifteen months I am completely free from pain and I shall be forever grateful to you for what you have done. Thanking you once again and wishing you all the best – Mrs W.'

As I go through these case histories I feel that I have gained a lot of experience of life, through the experiences of my patients. I am learning that the true object of life is that mankind should attain wisdom through experience. This cannot be accomplished by giving in to the difficulties of life but only by overcoming them. I have come to believe that the promises of God are not made to those who fail in life's battle, but to those who 'overcome'.

It seems to me that most people seek an easy life, a good time and freedom from care and suffering. But, in spite of all their seeking, they can never find that which they desire. People who think that they can go through life with no unpleasant experiences, trials, difficulties or adversities are chasing rainbows – there is no such thing as an easy life. The only life that is worthwhile is the life of the strong soul who has overcome. It is impossible to have an easy life and, in my opinion, if it were possible life would not be worth living, for the sole object of life is the building of character.

I never cease to wonder at the strength of mind and character shown by so many of my patients, the trials and adversities that they overcome, and the cheerfulness with which they bear the excruciating pain of arthritis. So many people, the elderly especially, turn to prayer in their suffering and many tell me that it was the Lord who led them to contact me. These people can't lose no matter how long it takes them to clear themselves of their pain. They come to the clinic so cheerful, so confident and so willing to do anything to achieve peace of mind and body. In my opinion, success depends on faith in God, and I feel so privileged to be allowed to glimpse into the lives of so many people and help them to overcome some of their sufferings. What a privilege this is – it has taught me so many lessons.

Case History 4 – Mr F

The following is the story of a young man of 40 years of age, with a young family, whose wife wrote the following letter to us on April 11th 1988:

Dear Nurse Hills,

My husband who is just 40, has recently been diagnosed as having rheumatoid arthritis. Wanting to know as much as possible about this condition we bought your book 'Curing Arthritis – The Drug-Free Way'. We were greatly encouraged by what we read and embarked upon your regime straight away. We have both adopted a positive frame of mind and are determined to cure this disease.

I am alarmed, to say the least, at how rapidly this illness is affecting my husband. He appears to have become an old man in a matter of weeks and is sometimes extremely uncomfortable with a lot of pain and discomfort. He obviously has to continue with his job as best he can (he is an estate agent). We are expecting a baby next month and one of our children is handicapped so I am sure you must understand how important it is for him to get better.

I realize it is difficult for you to answer individual queries but perhaps you could just let us know if he is hampering your regime by taking prescribed drugs for the condition. At the moment he takes 2 Indomethacin a day, and 2 Co-proximal when the pain is really bad. He usually manages with 4–6 in 24 hours. He has also been prescribed Salazopyrin but has not started to take these as we would prefer your drug-free treatment. He would adhere to this to the letter. We would really appreciate your comments and also any up to date information you may have. Thank you so much for the help you have already given through your book. Yours sincerely, SF.

Having read the above letter we sent Mr F our usual question-naire which he filled in and returned to us. He stated that he was losing sleep, had a lot of pain, was excessively tired and very depressed. He also stated that he was taking Indomethacin and Distalgesic.

We decided that because he was on Indomethacin and Distalgesic (a very strong painkiller) and because of his sleepless-ness, pain, tiredness and depression, that a urine and blood pressure test would be necessary. We also wanted to test for calcium, iron and zinc, so we invited him for a consultation on April 29th 1988, which he readily accepted.

During our consultation he told me he had been attending the hospital since September 1987 but that his condition was rapidly getting worse. His wife had to help him upstairs, it was a struggle for him to use the gear stick in his car – in fact everything was becoming too much for him.

A urine examination showed very high acids. He told me that he had seen his consultant three weeks previously as his throat had been very inflamed. This consultant had put him on Indomethacin and Distalgesic. Previously his consultant had given him 500 mg Naprosyn, but that had done no good.

On examination we found that Mr F's immune system was very low – drugs can drain the immune system. To counteract that condition we advised him to take Zinc (see Chapter 4).

Indomethacin can have very severe side effects including: headaches; dizziness and light-headedness; ulceration and bleeding; occasionally some drowsiness; mental confusion; depression; fainting; blood disorders; hypertension; hyper-glycaemia; blurred vision; corneal deposits; and peripheral neuropathy. Our first thought was, therefore, to help Mr F gradually cut out that drug. This we always do with the help of DLPA – a strong natural pain blocker. The effects and benefits of DLPA will be enlarged upon in Chapter 5. We supplied Mr F with our acid removing treatment and diet sheet, explaining in detail why the offending acids had built up in his body, what to do about them and what to expect as he went through the programme. We advised him on how to cut down and eventually cut out his Indomethacin and advised him to come back in two months for another appointment.

When Mr F arrived for his appointment on June 23rd 1988, he

was delighted to tell us that he had completely discontinued his Indomethacin. He had had quite a flare-up of pain and stiffness, but we told him to expect that, because the drug was no longer suppressing the pain – it was now leaving his body naturally. He said that he was quite happy to take our advice, and we made a further appointment in three months' time.

Mr F arrived again on September 27th 1988, and what a happy smiling man came into the clinic. He had experienced no flare-ups of pain in the intervening three months and was sure he was on the mend. He produced a letter from the consultant at the hospital written on July 1st 1988. It read as follows:

Dear Mr F,
Further to your consultation I write to let you know that your blood count was largely unchanged from that taken in March. The inflammation index (ESR) that we measure in your blood is now 80 having been 71. This amount of variation is merely due to laboratory variation in measurement on different occasions. Best Wishes.

This really was a very high ESR reading. When it was taken he had only been on our treatment for two months and, of course, it was very early days – our treatment hadn't had time to work. He continued with our treatment and advice for six months. At his next appointment told us that he had an appointment with the consultant at the hospital, and he asked if he should keep it. Our reply was: 'Yes, of course', as any blood tests or X-rays should now show a marked improvement, and confirm for us that we are on the right lines. Mr F had improved a great deal. However, imagine our delight when Mr F received the result of his blood test from his consultant. It read like this:

Dear Mr F,
I am sure you will be delighted to know that your ESR reading (the level of inflammation in the blood) is now 3 having been 80. Perhaps I should give up conventional medicine and take cider vinegar for the rest of my life!

Mr F has now been discharged from that hospital as clear of

arthritis. He still continues to take his Margaret Hills treatment – his faith in it has been rewarded.

What a lovely story to tell – once again our treatment has been instrumental in restoring health and lifting somebody up from the depths of despair. Nobody, but Mr F, his wife and family can truly appreciate what this has meant in their lives. We have gained the trust of our patient, but have also gained a family of friends in whom we take a big interest.

The story above is only one of many similar stories that I could relate. Consultants in many hospitals see the results of my treatment. They see their patients improving so much they can't believe it. They are amazed that it is all achieved without the aid of devastating drugs. Many patients are frightened to tell their consultants that they are taking my treatment, because many consultants and doctors do not appreciate the most important thing of all – that is treating the person as a whole instead of treating symptoms. We have ear, nose and throat specialists, chest specialists – all sorts of specialists. But it has been proved to me time after time that what happens in the digestive system has a direct bearing on the stomach, intestines, chest, ear, nose, throat in fact on all the systems, including, of course, the nervous system, and the muscles and joints. We should pay great attention to what we put into our mouths. Gentle, natural treatment takes a long time to work but in the long run the patient emerges as a happy, healthy person.

Case History 5 – Mr B

Mr B arrived for an appointment on April 12th 1985. He was 35 years of age. He had his own building business and was very frightened that he would have to give it up because of the pain in his right hip and left knuckle and thumb. He also had a tennis elbow. He has two children.

He told me that someone had photocopied my diet for him and that he had been on this for six months, but instead of feeling better he actually felt worse. On examination I found he had a marked lack of zinc and calcium. This I expected because for six months he had been following the diet but not taking the vitamins, minerals or protein needed to replace those withdrawn from the diet, because they produce uric acid in the body.

41

We did a urine test and, apart from the large amounts of acid, no other abnormality was discovered. His blood pressure was normal. We gave him the standard Margaret Hills Formula and Protein with the addition of calcium and zinc. We also put him on the acid removing treatment and the acid free diet and made a further appointment for May 14th 1985.

When he arrived we did the usual urine, blood pressure, iron, calcium and zinc tests. There was very little obvious change. He related that he had more energy, more strength in his hands, and less pain. He had experienced little pain in his right hip and his left knuckle and thumb were less painful, he said he was very happy with how things were going. Another appointment was made for June 15th 1985.

This time he reported he was still very happy – he had lost weight, which he needed to do anyway, and was feeling great although his tennis elbow had flared up after fishing. He said he suffered badly with cold hands and cold feet. On examination we found a marked improvement in his calcium and zinc levels and we decided he no longer needed to take these. At this point we changed his monthly appointments to 3 monthly appointments. His next appointment was September 10th 1985.

At this stage he was very much improved, but his cold hands and feet persisted. For this we gave him extra Vitamin E, to promote circulation in these areas. When he arrived for his next appointment on January 2nd 1986 he told me that he'd had a flare up of arthritis. This is always expected, as it is only through unsuppressed inflammation that the body rids itself of arthritis. Mr B had had a bout of bronchitis and the left side of his neck had become swollen and painful. On examination we found he was quite low in zinc. This told us his immune system was under nourished, so we put him back on zinc for another two months.

At the end of that time Mr B's arthritis and zinc and calcium deficiency had completely cleared up. Since then he has taken the reduced nutrition recommended, and has led a full and happy life.

On one of his final appointments at the clinic he said: 'I feel better than I've felt for years. In my opinion the only healthy people in this country will be those who have had arthritis and come to you for treatment'.

Case History 6 – Mrs B

A lot of the patients I treat are on steroids, and Mrs B was one of these.

She first attended this clinic on August 21st 1984. She was 54 years of age, and a lovely lady. She told me that she had been in a car accident the previous Christmas. She had suffered a 'wrenched' neck, and the following March had developed widespread pain in her neck. Her GP had sent her to see the rheumatology consultant at hospital who did a blood test and X-rays, and decided to give her a Cortisone injection. She was also prescribed 7 Prednisolone tablets daily. These had very little effect and in June she was admitted to hospital for more blood tests. Physiotherapy was tried and another Cortisone injection – she was also given Feldene to take.

When she arrived at the clinic she had to be helped from the car. She had lost a lot of weight and was in constant pain. Her blood pressure was high, and the tips of her fingers were blue – her circulation was very poor. She also showed a severe lack of calcium. She told me her husband had to turn her over in bed at night and she sat in a chair all day waiting for him to come home from work so that he could put her to bed. To make matters worse her sister had died of arthritis three years previously and she thought she was going the same way.

Many people have seen a friend, neighbour or relative suffer with arthritis, and been aware of the devastation of mind and body to which they have been subjected. The prospect of the same things happening to them naturally frightens them.

Mrs B related all her fears and frustrations, and the stress produced as a result of these was, of course, adding to her condition.

I feel very strongly that time spent with such a patient is time well spent, as we shall see later in her history. I spent about 1½ hours with Mrs B, counselling her on the reason that she had arthritis, what we could do about it, and how we proposed to proceed. We find that our patients are very sensible, and understanding of their condition. We tell them exactly what we find and how we are going to treat our findings, and they are delighted to cooperate with us in promoting their good health. We advise them and provide them with the nutritional formula to carry out our advice, but the real work has to be done by the patients themselves. If they do not follow the programme of treatment properly, they waste their time and money, and our time.

On the other hand, the sense of achievement experienced by those who adhere to the rules and rid themselves of their arthritis has to be seen to be believed. Patients have blood tests done at the hospital that show them to be free of arthritis. Their emotions often overwhelm them, and sometimes they burst into tears of joy in the clinic. One patient recently cried at the thought of cutting out her Prednisolone and being a 'free spirit' once more. Of course we are delighted when our patients get a clear bill of health and are discharged from the hospital. Then we have another success story to add to our list.

On September 19th 1985 Mrs B had a second appointment. She told us that she had done everything we had told her to do, such as reducing her Prednisolone gradually, with the back up of the treatment we had given her. She said she had a very bad time. This was to be expected because of decreasing the Prednisolone. She said she was having hydrotherapy at the hospital – I feel this is a very good treatment and always encourage it. On taking Mrs B's blood pressure we found it to be very high. She said she felt very light-headed. She was not menopausal, as her menopause had finished seven years previously. We asked her to carry on the treatment as before, but added Lecithin for high blood pressure. During the following month Mrs B cut out all her drugs completely. This is something I would not advise a patient to do. I always advise cutting drugs out gradually. However, Mrs B said they did no good anyway and that the side effects, for example, high blood pressure, light-headedness and poor circulation, were beginning to take their toll. This frightened Mrs B and she decided to drop her drugs altogether. She related to me during this appointment that she was now getting out of bed unaided, taking no drugs at all, and walking much better, with no pain.

She showed lack of circulation in her right hand and the toes of her right foot. She also showed a lack of iron. We gave her iron plus Vitamin C to absorb it, and Vitamin E to promote circulation in her hand and toes. She said she was due for an appointment with the consultant at the hospital. When she told him that she was not taking drugs he was not amused and put her back on steroids, which she refused to take. She continued to take the medication we had prescribed for her and continued to achieve good results, although she did have set backs (flare-ups) from time to time.

When Mrs B attended for an appointment on December 11th 1985 she said she was feeling much better, but that she did not sleep very well. To correct this situation we gave her Vitamin B complex to feed her nerves, and asked her to take her Protein in the evening. Her iron deficiency had now cleared up and she was beginning to feel very well. She said she can now turn over in bed without pain and do most things for herself – she was getting her strength back in her hands. Time went by and every day brought improvement to Mrs B, until on May 7th 1986 she arrived for an appointment telling me that she was feeling on top of the world. She was then discharged from the clinic but continued to follow all instructions and kept on taking a full quota of nutrition for another six months, to make sure that all was well.

Now, four years later Mrs B is well enough to hold down a very demanding job, which she has been doing for some time.

Every patient differs in lifestyle, emotions, fears, and frustrations. Some are coping with divorce, some with bereavement, some are trying to cope with an unruly son or daughter, others are wrestling with the stresses and strains of their jobs. The list is endless. Every facet of these peoples' lives must be taken into consideration in an attempt to alleviate the stress involved. They need constant encouragement and sometimes a little chivvying. Most of them need a lot of sympathy and empathy to help them through their particular crises. We always feel that a tremendous honour has been bestowed upon us in being allowed to help others in this way. Every patient needs individual treatment and we get a lot of satisfaction when we learn that a patient has overcome another hurdle.

Case History 7 – Mr M

On June 20th 1988 we had the following letter from Mr M:

Dear Mrs Hills,
Since I came to see you two years ago I can say that I have gradually improved until today I am practically a new man.

I stopped taking prescribed medication over a year ago and since then my condition has improved dramatically.

I can now crouch down and have had no trouble with my knees for months. I've had no pain or swelling in my ankles for equally as long. I now have mobility in all my toes and have had no back pain for a long time.

I have started playing golf over the past three months, something which I thought I would never be able to do again. Please can you tell me if I need to continue with the Formula on a daily basis. Thank you for your help in returning me to pain-free mobility which is almost miraculous – Yours faithfully.

Mr M had had arthritis in every joint of his body when he came to the clinic two years previously. He had been taking Indomethacin for years, and also large amounts of paracetamol. As he said in his letter, in twelve months he completely discontinued the Indomethacin and now he doesn't need paracetamol either.

In reply to Mr M's question: 'Do I need to continue with your Formula and Protein on a daily basis or can I stop taking it altogether?' we replied, as we do to all our patients who have got rid of their arthritis, saying that he could now discontinue his Protein, but that he should take a sachet of the Formula every other day, and Vitamin C on the days that he does not take the Formula. This programme should be adequate to keep the acids down, helped by a daily dose of cider vinegar and honey, and a good nourishing wholefood diet. We refer to this programme as 'maintenance treatment'. We anticipate no more problems with Mr M if he continues with this regime.

Cast History 8 – Miss B

Miss B was a 34-year-old lady when she filled in her questionnaire. She was getting quite a lot of pain and depression. She had had arthritis for 13 months. She told us that since the illness began she had experienced very poor digestion and an upset stomach, very often coupled with flatulence and diarrhoea. For the swelling of her joints she had been prescribed Naproxen by her doctor. On taking this drug the swelling had been lessened, but she was very troubled with muscular aches and weakness.

Having processed her questionnaire, we decided that she did not need an appointment and anticipated her getting very good results with home treatment.

On August 15th 1986 we wrote to her advising her to reduce her Naproxen in one month's time. We feel that a back-up of our treatment, for at least one month, is necessary to help people reduce their drugs. We sent Miss B our diet and treatment instructions, and also a supply of our nutrition Formula and Protein.

On September 19th 1986 we received a little note from Miss B saying:

I am feeling a lot better already and have less discomfort from muscular aches. My legs are getting stronger and I can walk quite well most days.

On November 15th 1986 she wrote:

My condition is showing considerable improvement.

Our patient continued to send in monthly for her nutrition. We wrote a little note back occasionally congratulating her on her continued improvement.

Christmas came and went and on March 17th 1987 we had the following note:

I have had a great improvement in my health recently, and the symptoms I was experiencing are now reduced to the occasional swelling, mainly in my knees. I have more strength in my muscles. Sometimes I have stiffness, but only in the dampest weather.

On July 10th 1987 we again received the following communication:

I have been following your treatment now for nearly a year, and have seen great improvement. Now I feel that the swelling and stiffness are linked to climatic conditions. For example, on a recent two week holiday in a hot country I didn't have any trouble at all, but immediately on returning to England, swelling started up again. In damp or humid conditions I notice the symptoms much more. But there are days when I feel quite 'normal'. Muscles and strength are gradually building up.

On October 15th 1987 the following letter arrived:

Dear Mrs Hills,
I should like to thank you for the service which your clinic gives. I have followed the treatment for over a year and have been free of pain for some months. The muscles of my arms and legs are stronger and almost back to normal. I was experiencing slight swelling in one or two joints when there was a change in the weather, but this is now just occasional and very slight. I am glad to say that I feel very well.

I should be grateful if you would send me some general advice on diet for the future. I would prefer not to take any vitamin supplements or special drinks if at all possible. I have changed my diet completely to take in as much fruit and vegetables as possible with fish as my main protein. I look forward to hearing from you and thank you again for your help and encouragement.

We replied in the following manner:

Dear Miss B,
You say in your letter that you experience swelling in one or two of your joints when there is a change in the weather. When you were on holiday abroad you felt no sign of arthritis at all. This is marvellous, but as we are approaching the colder winter weather now, we feel that you may be considering leaving off this treatment a little too soon. Whilst you still get occasional swelling, there is still acid in your body, and stopping the treatment too soon may result in a return of the arthritis, and mean having to start from scratch all over again. Please continue with your complete regime until January and if by then you have not had any signs of arthritis we will advise you further.

In fact Miss B continued to take her treatment until April, when she wrote her final letter to us. It went as follows:

Dear Mrs Hills,
I have acted on advice given by you at the end of last year and continued with the recommended treatment through the winter. It is now three and a half months since any of the arthritic symptoms have shown and I am feeling very well. My legs and arms are strong again and I can walk long distances and even run. Of course I am very happy and relieved to have a return of good health, and I would appreciate your advice on good dietary practice in the future. My sincere thanks for your service.

We replied to Miss B on April 6th 1988, giving her exactly the same advice that we give all our patients, that is to keep on with the maintainence treatment. Miss B has had no more trouble.

Case History 9 – Mrs S

On February 13th 1987 Mrs S filled in our questionnaire and returned it. She was a 54-year-old lady who was suffering rather badly with her nerves. She said she had some heart flutterings, and suffered from headaches, loss of sleep, cramp, pins and needles, and a lot of pain in her arms and fingers. She had excessive tiredness and depression. There were a lot of ridges in her nails but no white spots. She had had arthritis for 5 years but was not taking any drugs. It was very refreshing to find a patient who is not taking any prescribed drugs. We feel that our patient will get quicker results, because of not having any side effects to overcome. Having processed her questionnaire we decided we would start her off on the basic Margaret Hills Formula and Protein. We wrote to her telling her to let us know how she got on as she reordered, because if her symptoms did not subside there was a lot more we could do.

On March 9th 1987 we had a little note from Mrs S saying she was feeling better in herself and telling us that we had given her hope for the future. On April 2nd we had another little note saying: 'The pain and stiffness in my arms and hands has eased slightly, but some days it is worse than others. I still feel better in myself'.

June 4th arrived and so did another little note from Mrs S. This time it read: 'I'm feeling a lot better – sleeping well at last and having less pain'.

On October 5th 1987 Mrs S wrote the following:

I feel that I am now 100% clear of arthritis and I really feel fine. I will be pleased to receive your advice for the future.

We gave her the same advice that we give all our patients who clear themselves of that dreadful disease. We congratulate them and rejoice with them, wishing them good luck for the future.

Case History 10 – Mrs B

On February 20th 1987, Mrs B contacted us. In her questionnaire she wrote that she sometimes had cramp and also lost sleep due to pain. She also got depressed. She had ridges on her nails and also white spots. She also had varicose veins. She had first felt twinges of arthritis in 1986. She had taken no drugs. She was about 1 stone overweight. In addition to our standard treatment, which is designed to deal with ridges on the nails (lack of calcium) and all her other symptoms, we gave her extra Vitamin E for her varicose veins. Mrs B was 54 years old. We consider this to be quite young.

On June 1st 1987 Mrs B wrote to us saying: 'The pain I had in my hip is only a slight twinge now and I can lie on my left side in bed with no pain.'

July 17th brought the following note from Mrs B: 'I am feeling much improved, I don't get much pain in my hip now.'

On November 3rd 1987 we received the following note: 'I now find my hip is free from pain and my legs feel much better.'

We replied to the above note like this:

Dear Mrs B,
We are so pleased that you are now free from pain. Please continue with your complete treatment for the next three months and if you are free from pain and swelling during that time, we will consider you clear of arthritis and advise you accordingly.

Mrs B continued to send in monthly for her nutrition until February 15th 1988, when she reminded us that three months previously she had been free from pain and that she still was. Now she needed our advice on how to carry on.

We advised Mrs B to continue with the maintenance dosage of treatment. This she continues to do and is still clear of arthritis.

Case History 11 – Mrs F

On May 6th 1986 Mrs F came for an appointment at the clinic. She had been diagnosed with arthritis of the left knee, and degeneration of both hips. She suffered rather badly with her nerves, she lost a lot of sleep and was very depressed. The pain was worse at night, she had been prescribed Naprosyn. Mrs F was 56 years old. We advised her to start cutting down the Naprosyn in one month's time, and then gradually to cut it out altogether. This she endeavoured to do, but because of the pain involved it took her 9 months. By February 7th 1987 she had cut the drugs out completely, but was experiencing more pain. Her blood pressure was good, she was sleeping a lot better, but she was slightly anaemic. We advised her to take DLPA. This is a very strong pain blocker but also produced other benefits (see page 67). On April 28th 1987 we received the following little note:

> I have had four pain free weeks, which has been quite delightful. I'm looking forward to the next four weeks. Because of your treatment I am optimistic that I will continue to make steady progress.

Mrs F did continue to make steady progress and on September 8th 1987 she wrote the following letter:

> Dear Margaret Hills,
> I have been following your treatment for the past 16 months and have had no pain or discomfort for three months. Will you please advise me how to continue, and so prevent the return of my arthritis. My grateful thanks.

We replied congratulating her on her achievement. It takes a lot of perseverence and faith in us and our treatment to adhere to a strict diet and regime for 16 months. We find that when people see even a slight improvement in their condition it gives them encouragement to stick with it.

On September 14th 1987 we advised her to continue with maintenance treatment for the duration of her life. She has had no more trouble.

In 1986, BBC 2 came to the clinic and interviewed some of my patients. They were very impressed with the results that my patients had achieved. One, Mrs A (see below) had avoided a hip operation and was very happy to relate that when her hip was X-rayed at the hospital no arthritis was found. Several other patients also had very positive stories to tell, for example, one lady had cleared herself of arthritis in six months, and this was just after she had retired.

On looking through my case notes it amazes me how many patients have returned to full time work – people who thought they would never work again. It really is most encouraging to read what people say.

As our last case history (below) indicates, it is very important that our patients carry out all our instructions both while they are getting rid of their arthritis and afterwards. If they do not continue to take the recommended vitamins and minerals to keep the acids at bay, these acids could build up again bringing a return of pain. The vitamins and minerals we advise people to take help in the alleviation of many symptoms, including stress.

Cast History 12 – Mrs A

Mrs A, who took part in the television programme, is one patient who did not continue to follow our treatment. Having avoided a hip operation and been pronounced clear of arthritis, three years later a return of Mrs A's hip condition was evident.

On August 30th 1989 we received the following letter:

Dear Margaret Hills,
I am reordering after a lapse of about three years. I have been so well, but now I find that some of the old problems with my hip are coming back. I certainly do not like it, after feeling so

well for so long. I hope you are well and keeping up the good work. I spread the word to everyone I come into contact with who have problems, because you helped me so much. Lots of people have commented on the television programme and I know many people have benefited from it.

Mrs A felt that stress had contributed in a large way to the return of her arthritis.

On January 16th 1990 she wrote saying: 'I am so pleased that I am feeling much better once again'.

The case history of Mrs A proves beyond doubt that if the acids are not kept at bay, through taking the recommended vitamins and minerals, they will build up and a return to arthritis will be on the cards.

In the years I have been practising many patients have returned to me with a recurrence of the same symptoms. Once they go back onto the full treatment, i.e. acid removing treatment, plus acid free diet, plus vitamins, minerals and protein, they return once more to good health. These people have learnt a lesson. They don't deviate again from the advice given. Their experiences also teach us a lesson, that is, that our treatment works, and even if all our patients don't get 100% clearance, they do report feeling better than they have felt for years.

We have to hand hundreds of letters from patients at various stages of the treatment. Some are from people who have been told that nothing can be done, but who are now completely clear. This brings me to Chapter 4 – *The Stress Factor* in relation to arthritis.

4

The Stress Factor

Stress is caused by a negative outlook. Disharmony with one's body or with the environment are major factors that predispose towards arthritis and other serious illnesses. We are all aware when stress levels are creeping up, resulting from overwork, financial worries, marital problems and the feeling that we are not coping with situations that occur in the course of normal day to day living.

Some degree of stress is beneficial, both mentally and physically. It keeps us on our toes, mentally active, on the move, developing ideas and solving problems. Without it we would become bored, lethargic, restless and unproductive. People have varying capacities for coping with stress. One person's stress is another's exciting challenge. But if the level of stress becomes too high for us to handle then our health, and even our life itself, is at risk.

Our world has produced very stressful situations. The structure of our lives, changed attitudes to relationships, personal finances, ambitions, job prospects or the threat of unemployment, and even trying to stay fit and healthy all add to the pressure, as we feel the need to keep up and not fall behind.

The signs of stress are very evident when we can't juggle successfully the various demands placed upon us. We start to find these demands unmanageable, they invade all facets of our lives, they dominate our thoughts and interfere with our relaxation and leisure time. Our dietary habits may alter, energy levels drop, and our general health, family and social relationships begin to suffer. Some people turn to drink, others smoke or suffer from lack of sleep.

Our concentration at work drops off, but we still attempt to take on more to make up for our inefficiency, only to get bogged down even further.

The more worried we get, the less we cope. The body produces more adrenalin to try to keep pace with the demands for more energy, and in so doing becomes depleted of important nutrients.

If stressful conditions continue long term they can lead to heart attacks, migraine, depression, stomach ulcers and other serious health problems. We should all watch out for the signs of stress – they include headaches, high blood pressure, insomnia, difficulty in swallowing, chest pains, difficulty in breathing, constant tiredness, being easily upset, sweating excessively, palpitations, loss of appetite and argumentativeness and irritability.

When the above symptoms are evident, we are at our most vulnerable, and then disease sets in. We have neither the energy nor the resources to cope with it – be it arthritis, cancer or whatever – and we succumb.

When you feel stressed, in a panic or unable to cope, the best thing to do is to stay calm. Ask yourself if the problem is really worth all the worry, and save your energy for unavoidable matters. Don't brood over situations over which you have no control, and don't harbour ill thoughts and grudges. Always think positively, never think the situation is impossible.

Zinc deficiency

Pondering negatively on stressful situations depletes the immune system because stress in general increases the loss of zinc in the urine. It is zinc that nourishes the immune system and an undernourished immune system is very far from being healthy. People who have either osteo or rheumatoid arthritis invariably lack zinc as shown by the zinc test we do in the Clinic. Usually 3–4 months on a zinc supplement corrects this situation. Cigarettes and alcohol both affect zinc metabolism adversely, as do the contraceptive pill, most drugs taken for arthritis, prolonged exercise, sweating and hormonal changes.

In my opinion, zinc deficiency arises from two main factors – our present day lifestyle and interference with food production. We are all individuals and we all have an individual response to the nutrients available in our diet. Some people can make good use of the zinc available in their diet while others eating the same diet may be going seriously short. The stress associated with ill health goes a long way towards depleting the body of zinc, because when a person is depressed and anxious they cannot metabolize the zinc that is available to them.

Zinc deficiency can affect the sense of taste and smell, and a lack of zinc can bring about lethargy and apathy. In stressful conditions, when zinc is lacking, peoples' responses and reactions become pretty poor. White spots on the nails are an indication of serious zinc deficiency.

Because we specialize in the relief of arthritis, we assume that our patients have undernourished immune systems. Through experience we have found that by putting all our patients on a good zinc supplement, they benefit much more quickly. In the past, through lack of experience, we did not do this.

Drugs are a common cause of zinc deficiency in the body. The biggest culprits are the steroids, diuretics and antacids (all of which are given in arthritis), and the contraceptive pill and any hormone replacement therapy drugs. Any acute or chronic infections can cause a serious shortage of zinc.

In this book I am mainly concerned with those suffering with arthritis, but of course arthritis sufferers also suffer from various other conditions, and we have found zinc to be of tremendous benefit in treating depression, skin eruptions, alopecia, acne, susceptibility to infection, and poor nail growth. If we suspect a zinc deficiency in any of our patients we carry out the zinc test.

The zinc test

The test solution is made by dissolving 1 g of zinc sulphate hepta hydrate in 1 l of distilled water. One or two teaspoons of this solution is given to the patient who is asked to hold it in the mouth for about 10 seconds then swallow it. Responses differ.

1. Some patients notice no specific taste, these are likely to lack zinc.
2. Others notice no immediate taste, but after a few seconds a slight taste develops described as 'dry', 'mineral', 'furry' or 'sweet'. This denotes a slight lack of zinc.
3. Some notice a definite taste that intensifies – these do not lack zinc.
4. Some notice a very strong unpleasant taste – these do not lack zinc.

Most of our patients lack zinc and the dosage needed varies from patient to patient.

Treating the nervous system and minimizing stress

As soon as the immune system gets depleted the nervous system is automatically affected. The patient becomes nervous and skin disorders may appear. Sometimes nausea, muscle cramps, leg cramps, numbness of the hands and neuritis of the extremities are experienced. In fact a whole host of undesirable conditions are evident. The fears and stresses of these conditions add to the patient's dilemma, and very often when visiting their doctor they are told 'it's your age' or 'it's all in the mind', and they are referred to a psychiatrist, very often having spent months, or even years on antidepressants.

A lot of my patients arrive at this clinic thoroughly disillusioned with the medical establishment. It is not easy for them to cut down, and eventually cut out, their antidepressants. They quickly get addicted to them, and are very frightened of cutting them out. The same applies to sleeping tablets. One of my patients has been on Mogadon for 40 years. It no longer works for her, but every time she tries to come off it she gets withdrawal symptoms, even though we try to withdraw it as gently as possible. The lady in question is suffering from the side effects of this drug – these include hangover with drowsiness, confusion, and dry mouth. She also suffers from rebound insomnia – even though she takes Mogadon, she no longer gets a good sleep. When we try cutting it down she gets no sleep and goes into a state of panic and anxiety, but we keep trying.

Vitamin B complex

We find Vitamin B complex invaluable in the treatment of the nervous system and for minimizing stress. To work effectively all the B Vitamins should be equally balanced and taken together, because the taking of any one B Vitamin by itself, ie B6, can cause a deficiency of the others. Vitamin B complex is a wonderful morale booster because of its beneficial effects on the nervous system and mental attitude. It also helps in the metabolism of carbohydrates, and in that way it aids digestion. It helps the muscles and heart to function normally. The usual dosage is 50 mg B complex per day but certain individuals may need more. It is most effective when it is formulated with antistress pantothenic acid, folic acid and Vitamin B12.

Smoking, drinking, alcohol, a heavy sugar intake, and the contraceptive pill all deplete the body of B vitamins. Cooking destroys B vitamins in food, other destroying agents are caffeine and sulphur-containing drugs. There are three ways in which drugs induce vitamin deficiency.

1. They impair vitamin absorption in the body.
2. They impair utilization of vitamins.
3. Many drain the body of vitamins.

In fact, a lot of drugs take more from the body than they give. I feel very strongly that the pressures of life today on the young and the not so young, on school children and from then on to the age of 40 produce much stress.

Aspirin is supposed to be the household wonderdrug. I don't suppose there is a home in the country without a packet of aspirin in the medicine chest. At the slightest sign of a cold we all reach for the aspirin bottle. But very few of us realize that the more of these so-called harmless tablets we take, the more the Vitamin C is drained from our bodies. Aspirin can also lead to a deficiency of folic acid, which could cause anaemia as well as digestive disturbances, and of course large doses of aspirin can cause ulcers or bleeding of the stomach. All drugs have their own set of side effects. Having said all that, I realize that the pain of arthritis is so excruciating that many of my patients would prefer to risk the side effects of these drugs than put up with the pain. In the years I have been practising I have heard many say that death would be preferable to the intense pain, and indeed I felt like that myself when I had that dreadful disease.

Sleep

I always think that if my patients can get a good night's sleep it makes a big difference to their outlook and how they can cope the next day, so a first priority is to help them to sleep, as this is so essential to good health. During sleep bodily functions like breathing and heart-beat are as near to total rest as they can be. Without adequate sleep the body's physical machine would soon wear out and mental and emotional processes suffer. The way we sleep – the position of the body and its posture can also affect the health of bones, joints and muscles. If we recognize that we spend about one third of our lives in bed we should realize that our bed should be chosen with great care.

With good posture during sleep, joints and muscles can recuperate from the wear and tear of the day. Without it, that wear and tear will go on during sleep and aggravate such conditions as osteoarthritis. Good posture depends on the position of the spine. The spine, or backbone, is a collection of bones each jointed to the next. It is these joints and the discs of cartilage (the intervertebral discs) between them that get damaged and worn out by bad posture.

The spine is naturally curved. A bend in one place (for example, to incline the head) will require a complementary bend elsewhere to restore the weight bearing line. The curves in the spine are important – they are meant to be there whether we are standing, sitting or lying down.

In sleep it is essential that the normal curves of the spine should be supported. Back pain, one of the curses of modern civilization, is often due to sleeping on soft and saggy beds. Surfaces which become dented by the body's weight do not allow the spine's curves to balance each other out. This can give rise to back pain. A sagging or unsupportive bed will dictate the body's posture, instead of adapting to it as it should. Support is best given by a soft surface with an underlying counter-thrust, which can accommodate and adjust to the changing positions taken up during sleep. So choose your bed with care. Make sure that it is big enough for whoever is going to sleep in it, and that it provides adequate support for the spine.

People are, on average, now several inches taller than those those who lived at the beginning of this century, and many beds are just too short for tall people to sleep in with comfort.

Bed width is of equal importance particularly in double beds. Each partner must have enough space to move without disturbing the other.

The height of a bed from the floor is also quite important, particularly to the elderly and infirm who may have difficulty in getting in or out of a bed which is too high or too low. So pay attention also to the size of a bed, and make sure that this is correct for your needs.

Even bedding must be chosen with care. It must obviously keep us warm and also allow air to circulate. Unnecessarily heavy bedding, particularly when it is resting on the feet, can lead to painful foot troubles.

Pillows too are very important for a good night's sleep. A thin soft pillow with the correct shoulder width for you and which discourages you from sleeping on your stomach is very necessary. Sleeping on your stomach puts pressure on your jaw muscles and also irritates the neck muscles – not only that but sleeping on your stomach necessitates putting hands under the pillow which may bring about waking up with pins and needles, maybe numbness or cramp because of pressure on nerves and blood vessels.

In my opinion a warm protein drink is very conducive to a good night's rest. Restful music can also help, and some people like to read before going to sleep. In my particular case I find a little quiet meditation on the day's happenings, some thoughts on how to put right any wrongs done and some night prayers, very helpful. I feel a clear conscience is the greatest asset for a good night's rest – no harbouring of grudges. Victory over sleeplessness, or any undesirable condition, is brought about by absolute faith, confidence and serenity of mind.

5

Questions People Often Ask

If uric acid is the cause of arthritis why are some children born with it?
I believe that children who are born with a body full of uric acid have inherited it from their mother. A mother who has suffered with conditions associated with an excess of uric acid, such as migraine, asthma, bronchitis or rheumatism, can easily pass on high levels of uric acid to her unborn child. The uric acid may manifest itself as arthritis or rheumatism in the child.

You say the food and drink I have been consuming through the years is the cause of my arthritis, so why doesn't my husband have it? He eats the same food.
Everybody differs. In my opinion the acids build up in the joints and tissues if a person does not have the necessary vitamins and minerals in the body to burn up the acids as they are taken in.

For how long do I have to take the vitamins and minerals?
Because you have a tendency to build up uric acid, a certain amount of vitamins and mineral supplements will be necessary throughout your life to keep the acids at bay.

When can I reduce the intake of vitamins and minerals?
When you have been clear of all signs and symptoms of arthritis, ie all aches, pains, stiffness and swelling, for three months, we consider you to be clear. Then we advise you to take a maintenance dosage of vitamins and minerals.

What is the maintenance dosage?
This consists of taking the Margaret Hills Formula (vitamins, minerals) every other day, in conjunction with 500 mg of Vitamin C every day. (There is 500 mg Vitamin C contained in the Margaret Hills Formula, so when the Formula is taken it is included. On the days when the Formula is not taken, 500 mg Vitamin C should be taken.)

61

Do I have to keep to a strict acid free diet all my life?
No. Taking one dessertspoonful of cider vinegar in a glass of water daily, in conjunction with the vitamins and mineral formula every other day should keep the acids at bay, and a normal diet may be resumed.

What if the pains return?
You will have to go back on the complete treatment.

Have any of your patients been back because of a return of pain?
Oh yes – about five or six left off the treatment too soon and had to start again. Then there have been a few who, once they were clear, did not continue to take the vitamins and minerals – the acids built up again and they had to go right back to the beginning of the treatment.

My doctor says diet has nothing to do with it, what would you say to him?
I would say that he ought to look at the relief my patients are getting through diet, with the inclusion of vitamins, minerals and protein. He would soon change his mind. I would also say that some doctors and consultants have seen such a change for the better in their patients, they have applied to us for treatment for themselves. A few days ago a doctor wrote to me saying that when he had seen his patient, who had been suffering from extensive osteoarthritis, he had been amazed at the improvement he saw in her since she started on my treatment. This is only one example of the many letters we have received from doctors endorsing the treatment.

What vitamins and minerals make up the Margaret Hills Formula, and why do I have to take them?
The sachet of vitamins and minerals that you take each day contains:

Vitamins A and D
Vitamins A and D aid digestion. Vitamin A can be very beneficial in the treatment of weak eyesight, night blindness and many other eye disorders. It is also known as the anti-infective vitamin as it helps to build up resistance to respiratory infections.

It promotes healthy skin, hair, teeth and gums. It is reputed to be extremely good in treating acne, dry skin conditions and ulcers.

Vitamin D is very beneficial when taken with Vitamin A as it helps in the assimilation of this vitamin, it is necessary for strong bones and teeth and it helps in the treatment of conjunctivitis. It also helps to prevent colds.

Vitamin B complex
Vitamin B complex is known as the 'morale' vitamin because of its beneficial effects on the nervous system and mental attitude. It too aids digestion, especially of carbohydrates. It restores sleep and feeds the nervous system so that pain is minimized. It keeps the muscles and heart functioning properly. It relieves post-operative pain. Smoking, drinking alcohol and heavy sugar consumption all deplete Vitamin B in the body, and if such factors are present, far more than 50 mg per day is needed. Pregnant and nursing mothers, and anybody taking the contraceptive pill also need more. People suffering with neuritis and arthritis get tremendous relief from taking Vitamin B complex.

Vitamin C
Vitamin C is wonderful in the prevention of allergies. It is also most important for growth and repair of blood vessels, teeth, bones and body tissues. It also helps in the absorption of iron. Smokers have a great need for Vitamin C, as each cigarette smoked destroys 25 mg of Vitamin C. Like Vitamins A and D, Vitamin C helps in preventing infections. It also helps in the healing of burns, wounds and bleeding gums. It has a very beneficial effect on blood cholesterol levels, and also helps prevent blood clots in the veins. Of course, as we all know it helps to prevent the common cold. Because the citrus fruits (the main sources of Vitamin C) are withdrawn from the arthritis diet, it is most important that this vitamin is taken daily.

Vitamin E and Selenium
Vitamin E prevents and dissolves blood clots, increases circulation and strengthens the heart and artery walls. It is believed to help to prevent ageing by retarding cellular ageing. It helps in the healing of burns, ulcers and scars, and helps to lower blood pressure. Inorganic iron such as ferrous sulphate destroys Vitamin E in the body, so the two should never be taken

together. A period of about 10 hours should elapse between taking these two. Organic iron (for example that derived from food) does not destroy Vitamin E so the two can be taken together.

Selenium helps Vitamin C, Vitamin E and Vitamin A to do their work in the body. It is particularly important that Selenium is taken with Vitamin E.

Iron

Most of my patients suffer from iron deficiency. The pain of arthritis drains the body of iron and of course the drugs taken for arthritis have a devastating effect on the iron in the body. Most of my patients have been prescribed Ferrograd, a synthetic iron. Some have told me that they have been on it for years but that they are still anaemic. I believe that synthetic iron is not absorbed by the body, because when my patients have spent a few months on my natural organic iron, in conjunction with Vitamin C, they seem to recover from their anaemia – blood tests at the hospital have confirmed this.

Iron is needed for the production of haemoglobin (the substance that carries oxygen in the red blood corpuscles). It is also needed for myoglobin (the red pigment in muscles). Iron is also involved in the metabolism of the B Vitamins. It helps growth, skin tone, resistance to disease, and also helps to prevent fatigue. The organic iron contained in the Margaret Hills Formula does not cause constipation, whereas prescribed iron does.

Kelp

Kelp is a safe and nutritious supplement which helps your nerves and muscles to function properly. It is made from seaweed and contains an abundance of vitamins and minerals. A lot of my patients suffer with thyroid trouble. Kelp has a normalizing effect on this because of its natural iodine content. Thin people can gain weight and overweight people can lose it with the use of kelp. It is very good in restoring a poor digestive system, is very beneficial in constipation, and helps to relieve flatulence.

Calcium, Magnesium and Phosphorus

Calcium, Magnesium and Phosophorus all work together to treat osteoporosis (brittle bones). A lot of my patients suffer with this condition, and when osteoporosis is present the skin, hair, teeth, eyes and nails suffer. This combination of minerals is extremely beneficial in these conditions.

Calcium Pantothenate
This fights infection, helps to prevent tiredness, and reduces the toxic side effects of antibiotics. *Candida albicans* is very often a side effect of antibiotics, especially if they are administered without Vitamin B complex. Calcium Pantothenate helps the nervous system, calms the patient and promotes sleep. Without Calcium Pantothenate the adrenal glands do not function properly.

Alfalfa
Biologist and author Frank Bouer referred to Alfalfa as the great healer. It helps in blood clotting and also in a variety of stomach complaints such as ulcers, flatulence and poor appetite. It is a natural diuretic and a gentle laxative.

The above list is what the daily intake of vitamins and minerals consist of. They are well balanced, compatible, and all work together for the ultimate good of the patient.

Why do I have to take the protein powder and what is in it?
We all need protein every day to maintain our normal bodily health – to repair and replace tissues and cells, and to build and promote healthy muscles. Protein is made up of 22 amino acids of which eight are essential. These eight cannot be manufactured in the body, so must be present in the diet.

Not everybody needs the same amount of protein. If you are healthy, the larger and younger you are the more you need. However, if you have arthritis or any other ailment, the protein in your body cells begins to break down, muscles become weak, energy wanes and you feel irritable and depressed. On the arthritis diet butter, cheese, milk, cream, beef and pork are withdrawn. In fact a lot of good sources of protein are withdrawn, so it must be replaced to enable the body to return to a state of health. If the protein is not replaced patients can end up worse than they were at the beginning.

Our protein powder contains the eight essential amino acids.

These are Phenylalanine, Lysine, Leucine, Isoleucine, Methionine, Threonine, Tryptophan and Valine. Histidine is also essential for babies and children. The powder also contains Vitamin B_1, Vitamin B_2, calcium, iron and phosphorus. It is a complete protein, containing all essential amino acids. Some of the amino acids have special properties:

Tryptophan reduces anxiety and tension, relieves depression, reduces pain, and induces natural sleep.

Phenylalanine promotes vitality and improves the memory. It is also an antidepressant, which reduces the appetite and can increase sexual interest. It needs Vitamin C in order to metabolize.

Lysine is needed for growth and repair, and for producing hormones, enzymes and antibodies. It helps with concentration, fertility problems, and in the utilization of fatty acids. It is very important for arthritis patients suffering from hair loss, anaemia, nausea and dizziness caused by taking nonsteroid drugs.

Methionine is a sulphur-containing amino acid. A lack of this amino acid can result in fluid retention in the tissues, and an inability to avoid infection.

All the amino acids work together to perform various functions in the body. The essential amino acids must be present in the correct proportions for the others to work effectively.

For people who do not wish to take the protein in powder form we have free-form amino acids in tablet form.

Protein and amino acids help to promote sleep. I had an old lady of eighty as a patient who for a long time could not get a decent night's sleep. Now when she can't sleep she comes downstairs, makes herself a drink of protein and then she can sleep round the clock.

You have said that I need to reduce my steroids and eventually cut them out – why?
The fact that you have been on steroids for a long time means that you have been on a very strong suppressive drug. Steroids suppress the secretion of corticotrophin and may lead to atrophy

of the adrenal glands, which can persist for years after stopping prolonged therapy. This means that your own immune system will not be able to cope with the pain involved when reducing the steroids, without a lot of help. When long-term treatment is to be discontinued the dose should be reduced gradually over a period of several weeks or months. The time period will depend on the dosage and duration of therapy. If steroid therapy is reduced too quickly it can lead to acute adrenal insufficiency, low blood pressure and death. Withdrawal symptoms may be noticed. These are minor and include rhinitis, conjunctivitis, loss of weight and painful, itchy nodules.

The side effects of long-term steroid treatment can be very dangerous.

What are the side effects of long-term steroid treatment?
The side effects can be very dangerous. They are: high blood pressure, sodium and water retention, loss of potassium, and muscle weakness. Sometimes side effects include diabetes and osteoporosis. Mental disturbances can occur particularly in patients with a history of mental disorder. Peptic ulceration is a recognized complication which could result in haemorrhage or perforation of the stomach or duodenum.

Do you think the steroids are the cause of my muscle weakness?
Not entirely. They may be adding to it, but arthritis is a muscle weakening disease anyway. Of course taking steroids which have that side effect only adds to the problem.

I do want to come off these steroids. What help, apart from the standard Margaret Hills Formula, Protein and diet, do you propose to give me?
We get all our patients off their steroids and nonsteroidal drugs with the help of DLPA.

What is DLPA?
It is an amino acid called *DL* Phenylalanine. It is a mixture of synthetic and natural Phenylalanine and it helps the body's own natural powers to resist pain without the use of drugs.

QUESTIONS PEOPLE OFTEN ASK

What can it actually do for me?
It is very powerful in the relief of pain. It can actually be as strong as morphine.

Will I get addicted to it?
No, it is nonaddictive. If you feel you don't need it any more you can discontinue it at any time.

Does it have side effects?
No, it is completely without side effects – it is non-toxic.

Will it interfere with my doctor's treatment?
No, it may be taken with any medication or therapy without adverse interactions.

Will I feel the benefit straight away?
Very few patients get immediate relief. Most of my patients need to be taking DLPA constantly (two tablets of 375 mg DLPA three times daily before food) before they get any noticeable relief. There are some who need to take it constantly for two months before they have the required build-up for blocking pain.

Is there any category of people who should not take it?
Pregnant women should not take it, neither should people with Phenylketonuria. People with high blood pressure or heart conditions would be wise to check with their doctors before taking it because it tends to raise the blood pressure. But I have found that this problem does not arise if it is taken after meals instead of before.

I become very depressed from time to time. What can you do for that?
I can give you Vitamin B complex. Two tablets of 50 mg B complex in the morning and two at night will feed your nerves, and of course the DLPA is a wonderful antidepressant. Zinc, too, has a very beneficial effect on depression.

How will I feel when my nerves are fed?
You won't feel so depressed, you should sleep better and the pain should become less intense.

How long do I have to take all these tablets for?
That depends on you – how quickly you react to the treatment and, of course, how strictly you keep to it.

If I take these tablets – the vitamins, minerals and protein, but don't follow the diet what can I expect?
If you omit any part of the treatment you won't get very far, and you will be wasting your time and money. The object of the treatment is to get you 100 per cent clear of arthritis, but we can't do that without your help in carrying out our advice. You need to cut down, and eventually cut out, your arthritis drugs, take all your medication and follow the diet. The patients who go along with us 100 per cent get wonderful results – but those who don't we feel are wasting their time and ours.

Is there any time limit on the treatment?
No, a few patients do it for six months and become clear. Others are on it for 2½–3 years. It varies according to the severity of the disease, the length of time the person has had arthritis, the person's lifestyle, the amount of stress involved etc, etc.

Every winter I get very bad bronchitis and have to take an antibiotic. What do I do then?
A lot of people don't realize that the bronchitis they get is connected with the uric acid in their bodies, in other words with their arthritis. If you clear your arthritis you may also clear the recurrent bronchitis, so you may not need an antibiotic.

If I do have to take antibiotics for any reason what is the best thing to do?
Antibiotics do aggravate arthritis so don't be surprised if your pains become worse. However, if you must have them, take large doses of Vitamin B complex (100 mg twice daily) to minimize the chances of developing thrush – *Candida albicans*.

Why do antibiotics cause thrush?
Candida albicans was discussed in detail in Chapter 2, but briefly – antibiotic means 'anti-life'. Antibiotics kill off the harmful bacteria, but they are also apt to kill off the friendly bacteria in the bowel, intestine, and whole digestive tract from mouth to

anus, causing ulcers and unbearable itching from time to time. When the thrush infection becomes established it can take months, even years, to correct. However, when antibiotics are taken with Vitamin B complex the risk of thrush is minimized.

I have heard that Zinc is very beneficial – is this right?
Yes, Zinc is needed in the body for proper bone growth, proper sexual development, energy production, and nourishment of the immune system. It also maintains proper blood sugar levels and is necessary to the metabolism of Vitamin B_6 and Vitamin A. Excessive coffee consumption and high levels of copper, calcium or cadmium may cause low Zinc levels and as discussed in Chapter 4 stress drains the body of Zinc.

How do I know if I have a deficiency of Zinc?
White spots on your nails is a good indication that your Zinc levels are low. Then there are deficiency symptoms like loss of appetite, joint pains, loss of taste, poor circulation, poor wound healing, delayed growth, irregular periods, dandruff, impotence. Zinc deficiency can be a big factor in rheumatoid arthritis, because of the undernourished immune system caused by drugs and stress.

What foods contain Zinc?
Wheatgerm, eggs, oysters, nuts, sunflower seeds and wholemeal bread are all good sources of zinc.

Can I replace the Zinc in my body by eating these foods?
You could not possibly eat enough of these foods to correct a Zinc deficiency. For instance, eggs are a great source of Zinc but the recommended intake is only 3–4 per week. You need a good Zinc supplement to get anywhere. We have our own Zinc supplement which we supply to our patients.

I have lumps on my fingers – will they go away?
Once you start the treatment, they should gradually soften up and eventually disappear.

Can you tell me what they are?
They are acid deposits. As the uric acid leaves your body you will be able to feel them softening up.

Is there any way I can speed up the process?
Yes, you can do epsom salts hand baths two or three times a day. During each bath gently but firmly open and close your fingers for approximately 10 minutes.

The strength has gone out of my hands. Will the bath help to restore it?
Yes, the baths are excellent for restoring strength in your hands.

How do I do these baths?
You put 1 teacupful of epsom salts in a bowl of water, as hot as you can bear. Keeping the water hot, soak and exercise your hands for 10 minutes. Then dry your hands and wrap them in a warm towel for 5 minutes to allow the pores to close.

What can I do for my feet – my toes are affected?
The water you use for your hands can be reheated and used for your feet. Soak and exercise your toes for approximately 20 minutes keeping the water hot. Dry your feet and put on warm socks or tights. You will experience tremendous relief and increased mobility if you do this two or three times per day for a couple of weeks. As epsom salts are quite expensive, you may reheat and reuse your solution three or four times.

What do the epsom salts do?
Epsom salts are a tremendous drawing agent. They draw the acids out through the pores of the skin. The epsom salts baths of the whole body recommended in the treatment have the same effect.

Will you please explain what a flare-up is and why we get them?
A flare-up is a state of inflammation in a joint, or joints. It can also occur in the muscles or nerves. When it is in the nerves it is referred to as neuritis. A good example of a flare-up is the formation of a boil anywhere in the body. Consider why the boil is forming – it is because the body wants to rid itself of an

accumulation of toxic materials (uric acid). As the boil comes up to a head it is painful and most uncomfortable. The best way to treat it is by the application of moist heat through a bread poultice, kaolin poultice, or hot epsom salts bathing, to encourage it to come out. Eventually the boil comes to a head and breaks. We continue to encourage all the toxic material (pus) out and, when this is achieved, the body heals itself and we have no more trouble with pus or pain. If that pus had been suppressed into the body a much more serious state of affairs could have been the outcome. The patient could develop bronchitis, pneumonia, cystitis and even cancer because of the suppressing into the body of wastes that it needed to get rid of.

Arthritis sufferers have an accumulation of uric acid in their bodies. The body desperately wants to get rid of this acid, so it produces inflammation in various parts. This is what we call a flare-up. If drugs are given to suppress the inflammation the acid will not be allowed to come out. Serious complications are set up, which may not manifest themselves for some time. The drugs will cure nothing, and the patient has no hope of getting better – only of having lessened pain for a short time. As the uric acid condition advances, it gets worse. The body again tries to get rid of it and there is another flare-up. The doctor is called, gives a stronger drug, and tells the patient she has to 'live with it'. That 'it is her age' or 'wear and tear'. Many patients of 39–40 years of age have been told they have 'wear and tear'. At 36, I was told that it was wear and tear but here I am at 65 without pain and minus wear and tear – seems ridiculous doesn't it?

If, however, the acid free diet, with vitamins minerals and protein is followed, the acid-removing treatment of cider vinegar, honey and molasses is taken, and epsom salts baths are taken, the acid will be eliminated naturally by the body. This natural treatment was described in detail in Chapters 2 and 3.

It takes a long time for the body to get rid of an accumulation of acid, but with this gentle, natural treatment the patient emerges in better health than he or she has known for years.

The results of the foregoing treatment are a far cry from the drug therapy administered by the medical profession. Unfortunately many people can't afford the supplementary vitamins, minerals and protein and whenever we look in papers today the medical profession are protesting against them. They have completely closed minds. Those doctors whom we are treating, though, realize the benefits. Many have seen the results of this treatment in their patients but won't admit to the patients the reason for their well being – saying they would probably have got better anyway. But people are not stupid – they know the reason and tell fellow sufferers hence the reason that this clinic has become known far and wide.

When hands and feet are deformed can that be put right?
Sometimes the deformities are too great for the particular joints to return to normal. However, a certain amount of strength and movement is usually regained with the constant use of the epsom salts baths in conjunction with the rest of the treatment.

Why do you think I have this continuous ringing noise in my ears – I only take Brufen?
Brufen is a nonsteroid drug – it could be responsible for your ringing noises.

Does it have any other side effects?
Yes it does have quite an array of them. Namely: gastrointestinal discomfort, ulceration, bleeding or nausea, sometimes vertigo, mental confusion, hypersensitivity reactions (angioedema, bronchospasm and rashes), and occasionally oedema, myocarditis, and blood disorders (particularly thrombocytopenia).

Do these side effects apply to all nonsteroid drugs?
Yes they do, and recently it has been shown that osteoporosis can also be caused.

I know many hundreds have taken up your drug-free treatment but why aren't all arthritis sufferers doing it?
There are a lot of arthritis sufferers who are in too much pain to think for themselves. A lot live alone and haven't the energy to change their diet or to do the treatment.

There are also many who just get the odd pains and think it isn't too bad – they can live with it. Often though, these people realize that it doesn't stop there, it gets worse – very quickly sometimes. Then we receive an urgent letter for treatment.

In what sort of situation does arthritis erupt quickly?
Usually in stressful situations. Emotional stress usually aggravates the condition, for example, losing a spouse through death or divorce, losing a job, or having a family upset. Physical illness or an accident can also trigger it off. There are many stressful situations that can be responsible.

I broke my wrist two years ago, and since then it has been painful. Now my GP says I've got arthritis there. Was the accident the cause of my arthritis?
No, the accident was not the direct cause of your arthritis. A lot of people are misguided in this respect. Uric acid is the cause of arthritis. If you don't have uric acid you don't get arthritis. In the case of your wrist, when you broke it an alkaline reaction was set up at the site of the injury. Then the acids in your body converged on this alkalinity for neutralization. But if you didn't have a body full of uric acid in the first place arthritis wouldn't have set in there, or anywhere else.

I was diagnosed with arthritis two years ago but for years I had been getting odd pains here and there. Do you think they were part of it?
I feel sure they were. Arthritis is an insidious disease: very often it has been building up for years before it eventually manifests itself.

Is it possible to have arthritis of the muscles?
In my opinion what doctors call muscular rheumatism is deposits of uric acid in the muscles.

My nails are very ridged and break easily. What is the reason for this?
Ridged nails denote a lack of calcium, for which I prescribe my own Calcium Formula.

What is the Calcium Formula?
It is a balanced formulation of Calcium, Magnesium and Phosphorus

Why do I need all these?
Calcium works best in harmony with other vitamins and minerals, including Magnesium and Phosphorus. Vitamin D is also needed – this is in the Margaret Hills Formula. This combination should have a profound effect on your nails as well as your bones.

How soon should I notice a difference in my nails?
In about six weeks you should notice that they don't break so easily. You should also notice a difference in your hair. It should be healthier, and your skin should improve.

In what way will my skin 'improve'?
The skin on your hands probably feels very rough now. You should find that it feels a lot smoother as time goes on.

Why do you think my fingers get so blue and numb?
That is because you have bad circulation. Vitamin E and Selenium are excellent in this situation. You should notice a definite improvement in the next couple of months.

The skin on my fingers keeps cracking in the cold weather. What should I do about it?
Keep your fingers dry as much as possible, and put on Vitamin E and royal jelly cream. At night, having rubbed in the cream, put on white cotton gloves.

Shall I do the epsom salts hand baths for my arthritis while my fingers are dry and cracking?
It is best not to, as the epsom salts could irritate the condition.

Is there a cure for arthritis?
Nobody can claim to cure a disease. It is the body that heals itself. But many, many people, including myself, have got rid of arthritis on the Margaret Hills treatment.

Why don't doctors prescribe this treatment?
It is not available through the National Health Service, and doctors, who are trained in drug therapy and antibiotics, tend not to believe in 'natural' therapies.

What do you think of hip replacement operations?
When the hip joint has deteriorated to such an extent that a hip replacement operation is necessary, then I think it is a very good thing. Hip operations today are excellent, the patient as a rule emerges free of hip pain and able to walk.

However, this does not mean that the arthritis has been halted in the rest of the body. Unless the acid removing treatment, diet, vitamin, mineral and protein regime is followed, the other hip will probably also have to be replaced at some point. And the arthritis will travel throughout the body affecting every joint and muscle.

What is your advice to those going into hospital for a hip replacement operation?
I advise them to continue as much as possible with their natural Margaret Hills treatment. It will continue to remove the acids from their bodies and will help their immune system to recover from the operation. Any operation is a shock to the body and the Vitamins B, C, and E help enormously to counteract the shock and to help with recovery.

Can you take too many vitamins?
Yes, for example you get a toxic effect from taking too much Vitamin D. However, there is no need to worry about the vitamins contained in the Margaret Hills Formula. They are all natural, of the highest quality, well balanced, and easily absorbed by the body.

What happens in osteoporosis?
Osteoporosis is a condition where the bones lack calcium, they become brittle and break easily. It occurs mainly in women after the menopause, and in old people. Many old people with osteoporosis easily break a thigh bone or arm bone when they fall. When the bones are brittle they take a long time to heal and are apt to break again in the same place should the patient fall again. Also if a pin has to be inserted to correct a break very often there is no density of bone to hold the pin, and it becomes displaced. This is a very uncomfortable situation for the patient and creates a lot of problems for the surgeon.

You say that it is very important to have vegetables. Why is this?
Vegetables play a very important role in our diet. They supply certain elements that are absent or deficient in cereal and animal foods. From a nutritional point of view vegetables occupy a low place in the scale of foods, but nevertheless they provide certain elements without which nutrition and metabolism would be incomplete.

Vegetables contain fibre in the form of cellulose, which enables the bowels to propel the digesting food along to be excreted. In the absence of this fibre the muscular walls of the intestine have nothing to grip on to and the peristalsis becomes weak, resulting in constipation. The green cooking vegetables and salad vegetables are especially valuable for providing dietary fibre. Vegetables are also rich sources of vitamins which perform the essential function of linking our foodstuffs with the actual nutrition of the cells and tissues. The green foods especially prevent scurvy. Most of the alkaline salts required by the body are supplied by the vegetable ration of our diet and this especially applies to salts of potash.

What are salts of potash for? What do they do in the body?
These salts help to keep the alkalinity of the blood, lymph and urine at the normal level and in this respect they counteract acidosis. For example the ash of the potato and parsnip contains about 50% of potash.

Are vegetables fattening?
All the root vegetables have a fairly high calorific value. The calories are present in the form of starches and sugars, for example, the potato, parsnip, carrot and beetroot. People with diabetes, or who are overweight, should only eat a limited amount of potatoes, parsnip, carrot and beetroot. Uncooked salad vegetables, however, are not at all fattening. One of the hopeful signs of health progress in the present day is the growing demand for vegetarian dishes. This demand has led cookery experts to invent many new methods of preparing and serving vegetables attractively. Vegetables should form a considerable part of our daily diet. They are blood purifiers and without their help normal bowel function is debilitated, leading to problems caused by constipation.

How can constipation cause problems?
In constipation the faeces stagnates in the lower bowel, and this results in the formation of toxins. These toxins are absorbed by the blood and have poisonous effects on most organs of the body.

Why are raw vegetables better than cooked ones?
Prepared and cooked vegetables can lose many of their valuable properties. Boiling vegetables results in a considerable loss of nutrients. These nutrients pass out into the water and are thrown away, unless the water is used as gravy or soups. Steaming is a better method. This reduces the waste to a minimum. The common practice of adding soda to green vegetables in order to preserve the colour is to be condemned as it destroys Vitamin C.

   Vegetables should be cooked for the minimum possible time to preserve the precious vitamins. Using vegetables in stews, broths and casseroles is to be recommended as by these methods none of the vitamins are lost, and the flavouring properties are conserved.

Which vegetables contain the most vitamins?
Those that are eaten raw. They have a delightful variety of flavours and colours. Watercress and spinach are both very valuable, as are all green leafy vegetables. There are two varieties of water cress – bronze leafed and green leafed. It is beneficial in anaemia. In the old herbal remedies it was used successfully in the cure of ulcers. It has been shown to have definite therapeutic value in all sorts of debilitating conditions, particularly in the relief of chronic constipation.

   Fresh spinach too is very valuable and claims a high place amongst green vegetables. It has a high vitamin and mineral content, and has a marked aperient (laxative) action in the body. Fresh spinach is a very rich source of Vitamins A, B and C, while summer spinach contains some of the bone-forming Vitamin D. In minerals it is rich in iron, potassium, magnesium and calcium. It is a very valuable means of introducing iron into the body. It is a very good laxative and known in continental Europe as the 'broom of the bowels!' Dried spinach too is a highly satisfactory foodstuff, containing a valuable amount of Vitamin D. It is important that we include plenty of fresh green vegetables in our diet every day, not only watercress and spinach but lettuce, radish, cucumber and all other salad greens as well.

Asparagus, sea kale and celery are also useful vegetables. Celery may be served cooked or raw and is a very desirable vegetable. It is stimulating, relieves intestinal discomfort, is a diuretic, and is beneficial in rheumatic and allied conditions.

How about potatoes? Would you recommend them to be eaten every day?
Most people look upon the potato as just a source of starch, but it also contains Vitamin C and a large percentage of nitrogen. The most nutritious part of the potato is the layer just beneath the skin, so if a potato is thickly peeled the best part of it is lost. New potatoes need no peeling but should be simply washed and wiped. The soft skin is useful roughage and the inner nutritious layer is preserved. Even old potatoes need not be peeled. They should be washed in warm water and scrubbed clean with a hard brush. This method will not remove the protein layer. Scrubbing and then steaming the potatoes in their jackets is a very good method, as in most cases the skin is soft enough to be eaten and all the goodness is retained.

Potatoes can well take the place of part of the daily bread ration and, if served with fish, meat or cheese and a green vegetable, form a balanced meal.

I have diabetes. How will this alter your treatment for arthritis?
The only way it will alter the standard treatment is that the honey and molasses will have to be omitted. The cider vinegar may be taken in warm or cold water without honey, and instead of taking molasses we prescribe 500 mg Alfalfa three times daily. The same good results may be expected.

What is high blood pressure?
Many of my patients suffer from high blood pressure. The past 50 years have produced an upsurge of this condition, and I feel it is a direct result of the way we live. Excessive smoking and drinking, wrong eating habits, and prescribed drugs, especially those for arthritis, invariably raise the blood pressure, and, of course, stress is a common cause of high blood pressure.

High blood pressure usually shows itself in middle life. It is caused by a gradual silting up of the arteries with an accumulation of toxic matter, particularly cholesterol. The toxic matter is deposited on the walls of the arteries from a heavily toxin-laden blood stream.

The more the arteries are clogged with toxic waste, the harder the heart will have to work to pump the blood around the body.

High blood pressure and arteriosclerosis (hardening of the arteries) are intimately connected. Both are direct signs of a life spent at odds with nature's rules for sensible living.

The symptoms of high blood pressure are pain, noises in the head, irritability, dizziness, failing mental power and powers of concentration, shortness of breath, disordered digestion, various heart symptoms, and many others. Some cases of high blood pressure will have more serious symptoms than others, depending on the general health of the patient, and the force of the pressure exerted in the arteries.

All effective treatments for high blood pressure are constitutional. Drugs may seem to alleviate the condition temporarily, but in the long term they make things worse, especially for arthritis sufferers. For instance some of the drugs given for blood pressure aggravate arthritis and even though the blood pressure is kept at bay there is an escalation in the arthritic pain.

I have found that the treatment and diet that I give for arthritis also has a very beneficial effect on blood pressure. I also find that the administration of Lecithin 1500 mg per day, plus Vitamin E (400 IU) is very good. The Lecithin dissolves the cholesterol build-up that is clogging the arteries and the Vitamin E promotes the health of heart and arteries, and increases circulation. The amount of Lecithin varies according to the severity of the case.

What is low blood pressure?
Low blood pressure is a condition in which the heart's action in forcing the blood through the arteries is weak. It is a direct outcome of a weakened and devitalized system. It is not a disease, but a condition that can be put right by a good daily diet, containing plenty of fresh fruit and vegetables, and gentle outdoor exercise. A good walk every day is excellent and, being out in the sun and air wherever possible is also helpful. All habits that enervate the system, such as overwork, excesses of all kinds, needless worry, and wrong thinking should be eliminated as far

as possible. Vitamin E (400 IU), in conjunction with Selenium, should be taken daily to strengthen the heart muscle and the arterial walls.

What is Psoriatic Arthritis?

A lot of my patients suffer with psoriasis. It is the most stubborn form of skin disease, and is systemic. No amount of external treatment, in the form of creams or ointments, will be of any permanent use. The disease appears on the elbows, the fronts of the lower limbs, the scalp and the sides of the body. It is sometimes present on the backs of the hands, the feet and the face.

It consists of round red patches of skin covered with shiny scales or crusts which bleed profusely if more than the very outer layer is peeled off. The affected skin also itches a great deal.

The natural treatment for psoriasis is identical to the treatment for arthritis. It has been proved to me over and over again that psoriasis is closely connected to arthritis, and to a state of uric acid in the system. As my arthritic patients go through their treatment the psoriasis eases off gradually and a full recovery is usually achieved. Instead of using the drug-based suppressing creams given on prescription, I advise my patients to dab their psoriatic scales with diluted cider vinegar, allow them to dry and then apply Vitamin E and royal jelly cream. The reason for dabbing with cider vinegar is to give the skin an acid reaction. For psoriasis of the scalp I advise my patients to wash their hair with a good shampoo, rinse thoroughly, and apply a last rinse with diluted cider vinegar. Half a cup of cider vinegar to 1 pint of warm water is most beneficial, especially if the hair is left to dry naturally.

What is Spondylitis?

Spondylitis is inflammation of the vertebrae of the spine (ie arthritis of the spine). It may occur at any age in a body which contains excess uric acid, and responds very well to the treatment we give for other types of arthritis.

It is a painful condition, and takes longer to heal than arthritis of most joints of the body because the spine is so involved in weight bearing.

What is Ankylosing Spondylitis?
This is known as bamboo or poker spine. It is mainly seen in young men between the ages of 20 and 40. Unless treated early with a good diet, as given for arthritis, and manipulation by a good chiropractic, complete fixation of the spine could be the result. Even at a later stage certain measures can be implemented to help the patient to cope with everyday life and boost the immune system and the general health. The patient should be guided throughout treatment by a competent naturopath.

As I come to the end of this book it is my dearest wish that I have given hope to the many arthritis sufferers that exist. I feel that hope is a very important ingredient in the treatment of arthritis. Another equally important ingredient is faith – believe that it will work for you – go to it positively. Dogged determination, day in day out, will bring wonderful results, and always remember that the Great Healer is always ready to give strength and support in our daily struggles if only we will call upon Him.

Please take note that the Margaret Hills Clinic has now moved from Coventry to:
1 Oaks Precinct
Caesar Road
Kenilworth
Warwickshire
CV8 1DP